# Recognising Autism and Asperger's Syndrome

*Recognising Autism and Asperger's Syndrome* is an accessible guide, offering information and guidance, self-help and coping strategies and illustrated throughout with personal quotes, vignettes and anecdotes from autistic clients with whom the author has worked clinically.

The book captures the individual stories, quotations and experiences, observed in adult autism diagnostic services, woven in with contemporary research, theory and clinical insights. It outlines the history of the condition and the present criteria for obtaining a diagnosis. With exercises, tips, questionnaires, psycho-educational work and advice sheets, this new edition also elucidates the female presentation of autism that has attained significance in the recent times.

The book is deliberately aimed at a broad audience of people: those who have just received a diagnosis and want to know more, those who are considering seeking a diagnosis, family members, relatives, friends and clinicians, including mental health workers, psychologists, support workers and all those who work with autistic people.

**Trevor Powell** is an experienced clinical psychologist and author, who has spent the last 40 years, mainly working in the NHS, in the fields of mental health, neuropsychology and more recently, with autistic adults. His previous books include *The Mental Health Handbook* and *The Brain Injury Workbook*.

# Recognising Autism and Asperger's Syndrome

## A Practical Guide to Adult Diagnosis and Beyond

*Second edition*

*Trevor Powell*

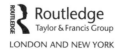
Routledge
Taylor & Francis Group

LONDON AND NEW YORK

Second edition published 2021
by Routledge
2 Park Square, Milton Park, Abingdon, Oxon OX14 4RN

and by Routledge
52 Vanderbilt Avenue, New York, NY 10017

*Routledge is an imprint of the Taylor & Francis Group, an informa business*

First edition published in 2015 by Speechmark Publishing Ltd

*British Library Cataloguing-in-Publication Data*
A catalogue record for this book is available from the British Library

*Library of Congress Cataloging-in-Publication Data*
A catalogue record has been requested for this book

ISBN: 978-0-367-42762-7 (hbk)
ISBN: 978-0-367-42761-0 (pbk)
ISBN: 978-0-367-85490-4 (ebk)

Typeset in Sabon
by KnowledgeWorks Global Ltd.

Access the Support Material: www.routledge.com/9780367427610

Printed and bound by CPI Group (UK) Ltd, Croydon, CR0 4YY

*To the children and their children: David, Marita, Tanya, Jonathan, Sarah, Hannah, Basti and Hannes*

# Contents

# Preface

Everybody is a genius. But if you judge a fish by its ability to climb a tree it will live its whole life believing that it is stupid.

— Einstein

This book is full of people stories, words, quotations and struggles; I feel very privileged to be a witness, translator and a messenger. I have tried to capture the experiences of autistic people seen in our adult autism diagnostic service and have attempted to weave the threads of their stories together to make a coherent colourful picture or tapestry.

The book is something of a hybrid, deliberately aimed at a broad audience: spanning clinicians who work with autistic people clients considering seeking a diagnosis, those who have just received a diagnosis, family members, relatives, friends, carers, mental health workers, social workers and support workers and I hope there will be some readership with the general public.

Helping people get a diagnosis can be rewarding, because the person has often been on a long journey searching for answers and is generally relieved to get a form of explanation. The diagnosis is often an enabler to acknowledgement and understanding and hopefully a signpost to further help.

However, there are a number of tricky issues in writing this book. First, the use of language and labels: whether to use the term autism, Asperger's syndrome, autism spectrum disorder, autism spectrum condition, on the spectrum, people with autism or autistic people! The choices are numerous and all refer to the same condition. Second, people on the autism spectrum are a very diverse group whose characteristics vary enormously, so not all the information in this book will be applicable to everyone. One autistic lady commented about the first edition of this book that that message, *'not all autistic people are like this'*, should be written in bold and at the bottom of each page. A third issue and paradox is that I do not want to 'medicalise' autism – it is not an illness. However, to get a diagnosis one is required to tick the box next to a number of 'symptoms' in a medical classification system. Fourth, I do not want to advocate a 'deficit/deficiency' model, but unfortunately in order to get help or *'reasonable allowances'* the person's differences have to be seen in terms of a disability under the Equality Act 2010. I hope that as a counter balance, I have acknowledged and emphasised strengths and skills. Addressing these issues is like walking on a tightrope. I have tried to be sensitive but know that I will inevitably upset some people. You are welcome to send me feedback.

For me personally, working with autism has taught me a great deal about myself. I came across people with autism in the later years of my career having previously worked in mental health, brain injury and neuropsychology. It strikes me that the adult autistic community is similar in some ways to the brain injury community 25 years ago – falling between the cracks of statutory provision, being poorly understood – a lost tribe. It has offered me the opportunity and privilege to meet a refreshing, honest, likeable and touching group of people. It is also given me a new lease of life and interest for which I am extremely grateful.

# Acknowledgements

I would like to thank all the clients I've seen in my work over the last 15 years or so. The stories have been fascinating and heart-warming and are the bedrock of this book – the golden nuggets. Their words and quotations have been anonymised in the main text apart from those who specifically have written pieces for the book in Chapter 4: Katie, Joanne, Rachael, Gerry, Floyd, David, Melanie, Julia, Max. I would also like to specially thank other clients Tina, Claire, Emily, Caroline, Rebecca, David, Jo and Felicity who have commented on my work.

I would like to thank members of my team and my colleagues in particular Ann Wilson, whose encouragement, insights and collaboration have been invaluable. Many thanks to other colleagues, including Georgie Boothroyd, Anne Jeavons, Andrew Salter, Sally Finnie, Maja Rogalewski, Hazel Kitson and James Jeffs. Thanks to Linda Bothwell, John Edge and Miranda Morgan, Sarah Powell for reading and correcting. Thanks also to Bridie McElhill, Dr Peter Carpenter. For the first edition, thanks to Bhishma Chakrabati, Jessica House, Marjolein van Deurzen, Helen Harris and Andrew Bates.

Thanks also to Professor Simon Baron Cohen for permission to use the AQ 50, Tony Attwood and David Lebond for permission to use the poem. Thanks also go to my employer Berkshire Healthcare NHS Foundation Trust, which has always been supportive of my writing projects over the years. Lastly, special thanks to my wife Meriel, who has given me long-standing encouragement and inspiration.

# Considering a diagnosis of autism

## Five people's stories: who comes for an autism diagnostic assessment?

### Jenny – 'it wasn't my fault'

Jenny sat opposite me in my consulting room, a single woman in her fifties, who worked as an accountant. Her face was rather expressionless, and her eyes flickered between me and the carpet. Rather directly, before I had finished introducing myself, she said, 'I think I've got a type of autistic brain. I want you to write a report to say I've got Asperger's syndrome, so I can tell my mother it's not my fault'. Jenny had seen a programme on television about autism, had researched the condition extensively and felt that it explained her lifelong difficulties. She had come to me for confirmation. She told a story of her difficult relationship with her now elderly mother:

> On one occasion when I was about six years old, my mother who was pregnant with my younger sister said to me in a temper, 'If this baby is anything like you, I don't want it'. That has always stuck in my mind. I know I was a difficult child, but what I want to know is, was I awkward or did I have autism?

Jenny gave an insightful description of how her brain worked:

> I have a brain that is attracted to detail. I love reconciling things – I don't care if it's a balance of one million pounds; I need to get it right down to the last penny. I am extremely organised and am a systematiser. My DVDs are organised alphabetically; my books are sorted by author; and my clothes are arranged by type and colour – although most of my tops are grey or navy and my trousers are black. My kitchen cupboards are sorted by food groups, such as Italian, Chinese, Indian, baking, sauces and tins.

However, when talking about her social life she commented,

> I have a small number of friends but I find meeting people is like
> going to the dentist – a necessity. I can never think of what to say and
> am never sure when it's my turn to talk. I always try and avoid the
> firm's Christmas party and on the odd occasion I have gone, I've felt
> exhausted and ill afterwards.

Another incident narrated from Jenny's childhood provided further insight
into her social difficulties. She told me,

> I must have been about five or six years old and I was happily play-
> ing on my own with my Lego and stuffed animal collection when my
> mother suggested I should go and play in the sandpit with other chil-
> dren. I said to my mother: 'I don't know what they're doing. I don't
> know the rules. I'd rather stay in and play on my own.' I remember
> her being angry with me and calling me 'awkward Annie'.

Jenny felt that her mother could not understand her and always thought she
was being deliberately difficult as she would only eat certain foods, didn't
like being picked up or cuddled and had to have things in a particular way;
otherwise, she would throw tantrums. Jenny did receive a diagnosis and felt
appreciative, tearful and relieved. I felt moved by her story.

## Stuart – 'an introverted introvert'

Stuart was 22 years old, with long blond hair in a ponytail, and was accompanied by both parents, who were sitting either side of him during the assessment interview. His mother said, 'I've told him he can't spend the rest of his
life in his bedroom. All he does is play on that computer, sleep and eat'.

Stuart mumbled, 'I'm OK, I'm happy, why don't you just leave me alone?'
The referral had come from a psychiatrist who had diagnosed Stuart with
depression, agoraphobia and social phobia. Stuart had left school with good
A-level results – A grades in physics and maths. He had started a course at
university on multiplayer game design but had dropped out at the end of
the first year. The academic work had not been a problem, but Stuart had
become increasingly isolated, finding social situations really stressful. He
had said to a fellow student on the first day of the term: 'I am an introverted
introvert. I do not find social situations invigorating like most people, but
draining … don't take it personally'. After returning to the security of the
family home, his parents and the cocoon of his bedroom, Stuart had become
more avoidant and further isolated. He would not catch a bus on his own
and wouldn't answer the doorbell or the house phone.

As a child, Stuart had been bullied and teased at school because he was
different. The other children would find his detailed and pedantic way of
explaining things amusing and would tease him in the playground just to
'set him off'. Stuart was like 'a little professor' and related better to people

older than his peers, preferring to sit and play a board game with adults. His father said, 'he never attempted anything unless he was 110 percent sure he could do it; walking, swimming and talking – everything has to be precise and just right'. As an infant, Stuart had started to walk very suddenly, in a very 'all or nothing' manner, with not much crawling or tottering. This 'all or nothing manner' was further illustrated in childhood when he told his parents, 'I'm not wearing a nappy anymore, I don't need to'. Stuart was bored at preschool because he wanted to do his sums and didn't want to play with the other children or draw; he had learned his alphabet before he went to school. He commented,

> I was looking forward to going to school because I thought I'd get an education. But on the first day we spent most of the time colouring. I thought this was ridiculous and felt disappointed and frustrated. I was more advanced compared to the other children and would go around the class helping my classmates to speed the lessons up. Towards the end of the infant school they took me out of the class and left me in the library with all the books and said 'get on with it'. That was great for me because I could study palaeontology and dinosaurs.

Stuart had been diagnosed by the psychiatrist with social phobia, but careful questioning revealed something about the source of his anxiety. Stuart explained, 'My anxiety is created by random events ... I need to have things planned; I want a degree of certainty; I'm afraid that if I don't know what is coming, I'll do something wrong; I'll create a problem; I won't know how to cope'. When Stuart dropped out of university, he planned to design his own computer games but soon realised that he needed to work as part of a team to do this effectively. Stuart's reaction to getting a diagnosis was a mixture of anger and relief. He said: 'If the incidence of autism is one in a hundred, why does it have to be me? But I suppose I am relieved to know ... it will take me time to process, I tend to keep my feelings in a box'.

## Lara – 'sensory overload'

Lara was a 40-year-old woman who had been arrested and charged with attempted bodily harm and assaulting a police officer. The duty court solicitor, who had a nephew with autism, thought Lara might be 'on the spectrum' and requested a diagnostic assessment. Lara was unemployed and lived with her parents. Every Tuesday morning, after cooking her breakfast, carrying a lunch box which always had exactly the same items in it, she would catch the 09.45 train to London, on her own, to visit the Natural History and Science Museums. She enjoyed examining the exhibits and making her own catalogue. Lara found the journey stressful as she didn't really like travelling on the underground, but she coped because she had a set routine and stuck with it, not liking change.

One day there was a closure on the underground and Lara had to take a different tube. The underground was very crowded, and people were funnelled, shoulder to shoulder, barging and shoving down a narrow concourse. Lara's anxiety, already high due to her change of routine, became extreme because of the noise, the crowds and the people touching her. 'Please don't touch me', she shouted out to a man pushing into the back of her. The man ignored her. 'Don't touch me, stop it', Lara shouted. She then turned and hit the man with a rolled-up newspaper, and a scuffle ensued. Lara tried to run away when they reached the concourse, but her assailant grabbed her in front of a transport policeman. The policeman tried to separate them, but Lara lashed out again, punching the police officer. Lara was arrested and put in a cell. She commented, 'I couldn't help it. I was completely overwhelmed, with the noise, the lights, the crowds, being touched, the change in my routine; I had a complete meltdown'. The man Lara had hit said that he would drop the charge if she apologised and admitted that she was in the wrong. But Lara was adamant that she wasn't in the wrong; she had only hit the man to defend herself after telling him twice to stop pushing and touching her. The man hadn't heeded her warnings. She could have apologised and walked away with a caution, but Lara had a very firm set of beliefs about right and wrong; she found it hard to understand others' viewpoints. Lara was later diagnosed with autism, and the accompanying report explaining her hidden disability provided more insight for the judge.

## Jack – 'needs an interpreter'

Jack was a 40-year-old IT specialist – a systems architect – who was accompanied by his wife, a social worker. He had come for an assessment because he was having difficulties with his manager at work and was involved in a disciplinary hearing. Their son Oliver had recently been diagnosed with autism, and both his wife and the diagnosing paediatrician thought Jack might have the condition too. Jack commented about his son's diagnosis, 'I don't really think there is anything wrong with him – he's just like I was as a child'. Jack described that in childhood he enjoyed lining up his Thomas the Tank Engine models by length, colour and personal favourites. According to Jack, 'My life was transformed with the introduction of the Spectrum ZX computer'. He said that at college he was rather isolated, having only one friend and no idea how to get a girlfriend. His wife, Sarah, commented, 'I noticed him, but he was hopeless and had absolutely no idea that I liked him, even though I was giving him all the signs, like always saving him a seat next to me at the Halls of Residence dining room – I had to do all the running'. Jack commented, 'Yes, Sarah has been a lifesaver for me. I would have literally been lost without her. She helps me with most aspects of my life'. Sarah commented about their marriage: 'I love him because he is unusual, fascinating and very, very honest and loyal even though he has an awkward disposition. There is no bullshit with Jack, but there is also not much overt affection'. Jack had recently experienced problems at work communicating with his manager, and on a number of occasions had not completed the tasks he'd been asked to do. Sarah commented,

Jack just doesn't understand what his manager wants; it's as though they both speak a different language, at cross purposes, which means the meetings they have are enormously frustrating. He needs very specific instructions - nothing vague. He might lose his job. I saw a sign outside in the clinic reception saying 'interpreter available' and thought, 'yes that is what Jack needs when he speaks to his boss, someone to translate and explain what each is saying to the other.'

## Emily – 'female presentation and misdiagnosis'

Emily was a single 32-year-old actress who had been seeing a therapist and psychiatrist for the previous 10 years. She had recently read an article in a magazine entitled, 'The female presentation of autism and misdiagnosis with Borderline Personality Disorder' and thought, 'that sounds exactly like me in every count'. At the age of 18, she had been diagnosed with an eating disorder but said that she was not obsessed with calories like the other girls and that her problem was more, 'selective eating and eating at exactly the same time every day'. She had later been given a diagnosis of borderline personality disorder on the basis of her difficult childhood, her stormy relationships, episodes of self-harm, sexual promiscuity and episodes of emotional breakdown that on two occasions had necessitated admission to a psychiatric hospital. She felt that she come to an impasse with the therapist over a number of issues.

Emily's father was a physicist and her mother a linguist with whom she had a 'stormy relationship' – her parents had separated when she was 10 years old. As a child, Emily didn't like being held and showed no element of fear around strangers. She was not a 'girly girl', but a tomboy who hated dolls. People were constantly surprised by the sophistication of her vocabulary. She reported that she had watched the film *Pollyanna* over 100 times as a child trying to work out how to be a girl. Emily had been to drama school, starred in a TV series and some films, but always had trouble with the social side of being an actress. Emily reported,

> The impasse with the therapist occurred in a number of areas, particularly with regards to the extent that I could change my life. I was not comfortable with being pushed to talk all the time, with the theory that the more I talked the more I would uncover some deep-seated trauma. I wanted someone to give me practical advice on what to do and I didn't want to desensitise myself to coping with social situations. However, the main area of disagreement was that she felt that I was the victim of sexual abuse, but I felt that I would often create situations deliberately. I was sexually curious and active as a younger child with older children. I also wanted practical help because I have 'an absolute inability not to tell the truth if the subject arose or if I observed an injustice'. I wanted to learn how to keep my mouth shut, be 'appropriate' and play the game like everybody else.

Emily was greatly relieved to get a diagnosis of autism and said that it helped her to understand herself more – she now did not view herself as being evil or defective, but just different. She found a therapist who specialised in autism and began to appreciate how the condition had shaped her life. Emily stopped seeing the psychiatrist and taking medication, saying she felt more stable. She reduced her sexualised behaviour, stopped her self-harm and felt more in control of her life.

## What is autism or Asperger's syndrome?

Each of these five individuals has something in common; struggles in life which eventually led to a late diagnosis of autism or Asperger's syndrome. Receiving a diagnosis helped each of them in different ways: Jenny found greater peace with herself, Stuart and Emily received a more appropriate psychiatric diagnosis and got more tailored help, Lara avoided going to court and Jack managed to keep his job. Autism is hidden, which is why it had not been identified earlier in those five people's lives. To all intents and purposes, the person appears perfectly normal, often very intelligent, living relatively independently, with near-typical language skills, but under the surface, there are a number of subtle hidden difficulties. These five people – Jenny, Stuart, Lara, Jack and Emily – are on the higher end of the autism spectrum, or scale, that is, they function relatively independently, while at the lower end is 'classic autism', a more disabling condition.

I have a clear memory of having worked with a man I shall call Lucas, many years ago, who had classic autism. Lucas had a below-average IQ with little speech and an array of repetitive stereotyped behaviours such as rocking, insisting on eating the same food and repetitively watching the same DVDs of *Thomas the Tank Engine* and *Mr Bean*. He lived in a residential care home, dependent on a team of support workers for many self-care needs. He rarely made eye contact but, when he went to the supermarket with his carers, he had a tendency to stand very close to strangers and stare at them inappropriately. He had no particular friends, apart from the care staff who looked after him, he had never worked or had a girlfriend. Lucas liked mechanical toys like Meccano and particularly liked taking televisions apart and reassembling them. In certain circumstances, he became very stressed and experienced what the staff referred to as a 'meltdown' when he would shriek and bite his hand.

What have our five case studies and Lucas got in common? They are all considered to be situated on the same underlying autism spectrum or continuum – illustrating how broad and diverse that spectrum is. All have difficulties with communication and in dealing with the social and emotional world, accompanied by unusually strong, narrow interests and repetitive behaviours. However, it could be argued that their differences are greater than their similarities. This is the debate that rages within the world of autism, between the 'lumpers', who say, 'It's all the same and we'll call it autism', and 'splitters' who say, 'People at the, so called, 'higher end of the spectrum', with Asperger's are very different and should be in a separate category'. There are arguments for both sides. Until recently, there was a clear division in diagnostic classification between people at the higher, less disabled end of the spectrum, who had a diagnosis such as Asperger's or 'high-functioning autism', and those people with below-average conventional intelligence, with more severe language and communication difficulties, called autism.

The recent American diagnostic classification, *'The Diagnostic Statistical Manual V'* (DSM-V), has simplified its diagnostic categories and reduced four subtypes of autism into one condition named autism spectrum disorder or ASD, getting rid of the widely used popular name Asperger's syndrome. The other classification system, *'The International Classification of Diseases'* (ICD-11), has recently followed suit, so it is likely that the diagnosis of Asperger's will gradually disappear from common usage.

A colleague of mine once worked in a school for people with Asperger's syndrome who were all very bright and often progressed to tertiary-level education. Five miles down the road was a special school for pupils with autism, most of whom had a learning disability. The Asperger pupils saw themselves as very different from the pupils in the autism school and did not like mixing. I recently attended a workshop on 'Communication Issues in Autism', by specialist linguist and author Olga Bogdashina, who has a 27-year-old son with classic autism and a daughter with Asperger's. She commented, 'I think it is a mistake for DSM-V to use only one category – my two children differ more from each other than their peers. My daughter speaks five languages and is at the university'.

The issue of labels is topical and contentious. Some people with Asperger's feel disenfranchised by the changes in DSM-V, saying, 'We've lost our label and our identity'; others proudly say, 'I'm autistic and proud of it'; still others say, 'I am not a disorder, I am not even a person with autism, I'm an autistic person. I'm not a disordered version of a non-autistic person'. A recent online survey of more than 3000 people, led by the National Autistic Society, found that there was no single term that everybody preferred. All groups, which included people on the spectrum, families, friends and professionals, liked 'on the autism spectrum' and 'Asperger's syndrome' although professionals preferred ASD more than the other groups. However, the current situation presents a problem for any likely author of a book on the subject – namely myself. This book is about, and for, people at the higher end of the autism spectrum in terms of independence, previously referred to as Asperger's syndrome. I will occasionally use that term, if that is the term client's use about themselves, but mainly use the term autism. Apologies in advance if causing any offence – there is no intention!

DSM-V suggests that autism can be classified into three levels of severity, depending on the level of support required. Officially, the people we see in our clinic can be diagnosed as ASD Level One, and add in brackets (Asperger's syndrome). The person must have had the condition since early childhood and there must be a significant impact or impairment on their life (relationships, work, mental health etc.). Autism was previously described as being a triad of symptoms, whereas the new DSM-V reduces this to a dyad, or two main dimensions or domains. These two domains are described in medical terminology as being characterised by persistent deficits in (1) social communication and social interaction and (2) restrictive, repetitive patterns of behaviour, interests or activities. Sensory sensitivities, which were previously just a footnote, are now a recognised as a full criteria, within Domain 2. Some people would view autism as quite a varied constellation of symptoms, which at first glance seem very disparate. To get a feel of the condition, I will describe the most common traits in each dimension. It would be useful to bear in mind that a person does not have to have all those traits to obtain a diagnosis.

(a) *Social and communication difficulties*

- May find it difficult to communicate in a two-way backward and forward conversation and struggle with making small talk.

- May have a literal interpretation of language – difficulty understanding nuances, jokes, sarcasm.

- Have difficulty understanding and using a range of non-verbal behaviours, such as tone of voice, body language, gestures and facial expression.

- Struggle establishing and maintaining relationships and friendships.

- Have difficulties recognising people's feelings or expressing their own.

- Struggle to understand 'social rules', often being too honest, direct or blunt.

(b) *Restricted, repetitive patterns of behaviour interest or activities*

- Having strong special interests that are often very intense or focused.

- Having a strong need to stick to the familiar – finding change and unexpected situations stressful.

- A good eye for detail, but difficulty multitasking and seeing the overall picture.

- Having certain sensory sensitivities around touch, textures, loud noises, tastes, smells, light etc.

- Sometimes having unusual speech or physical motor mannerisms, e.g. rocking, stimming etc.

## A dash of autism and the rise of civilisation

From the list given earlier, it is apparent that autism can be a diverse cluster or a constellation of characteristics that co-occur. These can be a strength; such as great concentration, an ability to focus narrowly and resist distraction, specialist knowledge and intelligence, as well as difficulty in the areas of understanding the social and emotional landscape or coping with the sensory world. Throughout history, people with autistic traits have led successful, celebrated lives in the sciences, arts, business and politics. Civilisation would not be where it is today without the influence of autistic thinking. Allan Snyder, the director of Sydney University's Centre for the Mind, commented, 'Nobel Prize-calibre geniuses often have certain core autistic features at their hearts'. Hans Asperger, after whom the condition was named, said, 'It seems that for success in science or art, a dash of autism is essential'.

High achievers throughout history are thought to have had 'a dash of autism', including Albert Einstein, Charles Darwin, Isaac Newton, Hans Christian Andersen, Lewis Carroll, Thomas Jefferson, Wolfgang Amadeus Mozart, Andy Warhol, Thomas Edison, and Gregor Mendel (Santomauro, 2012). Who would have thought that Charles Darwin's boyhood fascination with bug-collecting would form the basis of the theory of evolution and tell us about our oneness with nature? Nobody could imagine that Albert Einstein, who did not speak fluently until he was 7, had no friends and rarely mixed with children his age, being described as the 'odd boy out', would go on to win the Nobel Prize and become the father of the theory of relativity? As a child, he was introspective, avoiding light conversation and eye contact, but when something caught his interest he is said to have had, 'the concentration of a watchmaker' and a 'laser-like ability to focus', according to those who have chronicled his life. As an adult in his university post, he was described as a 'confusing lecturer' and considered a shy genius, saying of himself, 'I'm not much with people'. He was known as 'old stone face', because of his lack of facial expression and became more reclusive in later life. He also had a 'lack of a tactful manner', a reputation for bizarre clothing choices and unconcern about his appearance – his uncombed hair a signature feature.

More contemporary figures include most of those people who were the founding fathers of computers, which have transformed our lives. One of the pioneers of the first computer was the British mathematician, Alan Turing, who during World War II broke the German Enigma cypher machine code, saving thousands of lives and shortening the war and who undoubtedly had a 'dash of autism', as seen in the film *The Imitation Game* (2014). Alan Turing was voted winner of the BBC's *Icons of the Twentieth Century Award* (2019) and now has his image on the back of the 50-pound note.

Ashley Stanford wrote a fascinating book entitled *Business for Aspies* (2011) which provides insight into the development of the IT industry in California. She grew up in Silicon Valley California and married a man with autism, who was an exceptionally talented coder and programmer and founded a successful IT company. She suggests that numerous successful people are often not particularly 'well rounded' but have focused on their strengths. She comments on page 23:

> When you look at the top thousand most successful people of this generation you find a surprising number of them with Asperger traits. … One of the richest men in the world was Bill Gates, a man known for having many obvious autistic traits. I grew up near Redmond where Bill Gates established the Microsoft Empire. Many of my friends and acquaintances worked for Gates in the early days of Microsoft's growth. The stories of his fits, rages, rocking, obsessing, stimming, flapping and irrational hold to logical structures were part of many conversations with friends.

Stanford theorises that of the four men who contributed most to the design of computer operating systems, three exhibited mild-to-moderate autistic traits. Those men were Linus Torvalds who developed the Linux operating system, Bill Gates who developed the Windows operating system and built the Microsoft Empire and Steve Wozniak who (along with Steve Jobs) developed the Macintosh operating system and built the Apple organisation. Perhaps the only one who didn't have autistic traits was Steve Jobs. Autistic or 'black and white', logical, binary thinking and the ability to concentrate for lengthy periods and have an attention to detail are an obvious advantage in the field of computing.

Temple Grandin, who has achieved fame and success as an autistic person, has written books and lectured on autism and is now a professor at Colorado State University, is also a living role model. She writes how she had delayed speech as a child, was taunted for being different and was the weirdo at school whom the 'cool' kids teased. But, she found a mentor in a science teacher at her school who fed and encouraged her hunger for knowledge and understanding. Her natural affinity with animals, in particular the cattle on her aunt's ranch, led her to becoming a successful animal behavioural specialist and designer of humane cattle-handling facilities. Over half the cattle in the United States and Canada are handled in the humane chute systems she designed. There is now an Emmy Award–winning film (Temple Grandin – Drama/Historical drama, 2010) about her life. She commented, 'After all, the really social people did not invent the first stone spear. It was probably invented by an Aspie who chipped away at rocks while the other people socialised around the campfire. Without autism traits we might still be living in caves'.

Recently, there have been a number of public figures, exceptional in their field, who have 'come out' as having Asperger's/autism in later life. Their stories illustrate that autistic characteristics can have its advantages.

The television wildlife presenter and naturalist Chris Packham, who obtained a diagnosis in his 40s, made a recent BBC TV documentary

(Chris Packham: Asperger's and Me, 2019) and talked about his early obsessions with wildlife.

> I've tried for 30 years to hide it (my autism) and now I want to talk about it… I don't have the need for social contact … people find me weird which is why I live in in a cottage in the middle of the woods with my dog. I experience the world in a different way – it's like a hyperreality, the seeing, hearing, smelling and tasting. This sensory overload is a constant distraction … When I was a child the depth of my obsessions was much greater than my peers. When I got into things, I really got into them. At primary school I didn't have a need for friends, there were far more interesting things going on in a dirty pond over the fence. I was enchanted by every living thing … my interests were overpowering- I wouldn't stop going on about stuff.

In sport, particularly endurance sports that require solitary, repetitive practice, autistic traits come in very handy. The elite cyclist Jonathan Vaughters, US Time Trial champion, says he was diagnosed at the age of 45. He reports that as a child he was geeky and bullied, which gave him the anger, drive and motivation to succeed saying:

> My best asset in cycling was my ability to push myself to an extreme … I love the time trials, just me, the sound of the wind, the sound of my breathing, a road, loneliness and pain. That sounds crazy, but what I remember most was the feeling that I wasn't at a cocktail party with eight people … It's amazing you can go through 45 years of life and have something that is your biggest asset, your best and coolest weapon, that is also your downfall.

Motorcycle racer and popular television presenter Guy Martin, who received a diagnosis as an adult, makes insightful comments about the advantage of a single-minded focus, in becoming a top sportsman. He also describes his tendency to be honest and straightforward, 'telling people how it is'.

> It's probably what helped with the endurance racing on my mountain bike … I'm good at getting my head down … I find it difficult being in a crowded room for more than ten minutes and shy away from social occasions … I call it as it is. If people ask me something, I tell them how it is and it offends a few people. I call it 'Honesty Tourette's.

In the field of acting, an ability to copy, mimic and imitate others from an early age in order to survive offers a ready-made predisposition to being an actor. Paddy Considine, the British actor and film director, said,

> Naming my problem has helped a lot … It's enabled me to make sense of things I didn't understand before … I've always struggled with certain noises, bright lights and even wallpaper … I got through with my

ability to mimic others and make people laugh. I have grown up observing, imitating and copying people. I've learned all my social skills, they didn't come naturally. … But I find walking the kids to school and saying hello to people harder than being on a Broadway stage.

Sir Antony Hopkins, Oscar winning actor, commented, 'Asperger's has helped my acting … I definitely look at people differently … to work out what makes them tick'. He was renowned for his ability to remember lines and in the Stephen Spielberg film *Amistad*, he astounded the crew with his memorisation of a seven-page courtroom speech in one go. However, the actress Daryl Hannah said that her autism made it difficult to cope with the social demands made of Hollywood stars. 'I never went on talk shows, never went to Premiers … these days I have little tricks that I do to help me cope'.

One of the UK's leading business figures, Charlotte Valeur, former investment banker and Chairman of the Institute of Directors, revealed publicly that she is autistic, to alter the perception of autism in the workplace. This hopefully will reduce discrimination and make disclosure easier for others. Ms Valeur, is Danish, a single parent with three children, one of whom has autism, says she was bullied incessantly as a child, didn't get on with other children, 'became a bit of a tomboy', and still does not feel comfortable networking at drinks events. She was however a highly successful bond trader and consistently one of the top ten traders. She commented,

> I was a bond trader and loved it. It was high intensity work, you had to be on the trading floor, hyper focusing on numbers for 12 hours a day … Being autistic has given me immense amounts of creativity, drive and focus… the autistic brain can be brilliant at finding new solutions … I can't be sure if I'm going to be discriminated against because of this. There may be boards who may not employ me, and I must be prepared for that.

Greta Thunberg, the young passionate climate change campaigner and activist, who recently spoke at the United Nations and was voted Time Magazine, 'Woman of the Year 2019', is autistic. Her single-minded clarity, sense of what is 'right and wrong' and strong sense of social justice shines out. But before getting a diagnosis, she suffered from bullying, depression and an eating disorder and, at one stage, selective mutism. Her supportive parents have noted an incredible transformation.

The Japanese creator of Pokémon, Satoshi Tajiri, is autistic – he collected bugs as a child and developed a game that has become a worldwide phenomenon.

## A brief history of Asperger's syndrome and autism

Examining the history of autism/Asperger's sheds light on the complexity of the subject. Eighty years ago it was barely recognised, but now it has become the most talked about and controversial diagnosis of our time. The term

Asperger's syndrome is named after the Viennese paediatrician Hans Asperger, who wrote an influential research paper in 1944. However, the word 'autism' originates from the Greek word for 'self' (*autos*) and was first used by the Swiss psychiatrist Eugen Bleuler in 1912 to describe the thought patterns of schizophrenic patients and their difficulty connecting with other people.

Classic autism was first described in 1943 by Leo Kanner, a child psychiatrist in the United States. He described autistic aloneness or profound lack of social engagement in 11 children who had great difficulty appreciating another person's point of view and at the same time were very literal and experienced great difficulties with change. The first case was a boy called Donald T, who was described as being 'emotionally indifferent' and having an 'inability to relate'; he had spent a year of his early life in an institution. Kanner referred to this syndrome as a form of childhood schizophrenia, saying that it was very rare and inadvertently caused by the parents because of their 'cold perfectionistic' parenting style.

At the same time in Europe, Hans Asperger made similar observations about a group of children, describing a milder form of the developmental disorder. Asperger described these children with autistic traits who had an IQ in the average range or above-average range and who frequently had very good attention and memory for detail, often being interested in acquiring unusual knowledge, wanting things to be done in the same way over and over again and being socially awkward or withdrawn. He referred to some of them as 'little professors', gifted, solitary, with precocious abilities and a fascination with rules, laws and schedules. Asperger, however, did not go on to point the finger of blame at the parents.

Interestingly, Hans Asperger appears to have exhibited many of the features named after him. He was described as a 'remote and lonely child', who had difficulty making friends, was exceptionally good at languages and was particularly interested in an Austrian poet Franz Grillparzer, whom he used to quote to his uninterested and exasperated classmates. His landmark paper was clear in suggesting that he was under no illusion that the patients were budding geniuses and that 'Unfortunately, in the majority of cases the positive aspects of autism do not outweigh the negative ones'.

It was Kanner in the United States who became famous, an autism celebrity, writing papers and books and giving lectures. However, he made little or no reference to Hans Asperger and did not cite his influential paper. The excellent book by Steve Silberman entitled *Neurotribes* (2015) traces the history of autism, uncovering Kanner's suppression of the truth. The baton for 'blaming the parents' and spreading Kanner's theory of toxic parenting was picked up by another celebrity psychiatrist called Bruno Bettelheim. Like Kanner, Bettelheim was a refugee from Europe – a concentration camp survivor – who emigrated to the United States. One of the books he wrote was entitled *The Empty Fortress* (1967) in which he described autism as an illness, 'a suicide of the soul', and described the mothers as 'refrigerator mothers'. How damaging and unfair we now know this completely misguided belief to be and how awful for the parents to be associated with this type of shame and stigma! Not only did he blame the parents, but also he suggested various therapies to attempt to rescue the child from this condition. These included hour after hour of psychoanalysis, or, worse still, different forms of holding therapies, where mothers were required to 'tame' their children by hugging them and staring into their eyes. Undoubtedly, many lives were ruined by this cruel misunderstanding and pointing the finger of blame at parents. Eventually, this theory started to crumble, and the anti-psychiatric movement of the late 1960s and 1970s began to produce evidence that the judgementalism within psychoanalytical treatments was often more harmful than beneficial. Leo Kanner was later to apologise, asking the parents to forgive him.

Studies of autistic twins replaced the bad parenting theory with evidence that autism had complex genetic roots. Research into the parents of autistic children showed that they were no less caring than other parents, and with the subsequent development of neuroscience, we now know that people with autism have non-typical wiring of the brain. We also know that autism is primarily a genetic condition and that both parents contribute 'risk genes'.

Hans Asperger's landmark paper from 1944 was brought to a wider audience by the British psychiatrist Dr Lorna Wing in the 1980s. Lorna Wing had a daughter called Susie who had autism, and she experienced and recognised how little support there was. Wing was the first person to translate Asperger's paper from German into English and give it a wider prominence. She argued that autism lay on the spectrum or continuum and that it was not a categorical condition, but there were milder cases or 'shades of autism'. In a lecture I attended by Lorna Wing, she repeatedly used the phrase 'nature never makes a line without smudging it – the lines are all smudged' when referring to diagnosing autism. She also famously said, 'When you've met one person with autism, you've met one person with autism', meaning that autistic people can be very different from each other. Lorna Wing began a quiet but determined campaign to expand the concept of autism, make it more understandable and to elicit more support and resources.

In 1988, the Hollywood film *Rain Man*, directed by Barry Levinson and starring Dustin Hoffman as Raymond Babbitt, introduced to a wider audience the special savant-like memory skills of some people with autism. The film was enormously popular grossing $355 million worldwide and winning numerous Oscars. It gave autism a considerable profile, and people began recognising aspects of themselves on screen. This gave a huge injection of energy to support agencies and charities in the United States and the United Kingdom. In 1994, Asperger's was officially added to the diagnostic classification, the DSM-5, as a developmental disorder. In 2009, the UK government introduced the Autism Act, which was the first piece of national disability-specific legislation establishing the terms and provision of care for adults with autism and significantly increased the profile of the condition. Now generally speaking autism is seen as a lifelong condition – a 'disability' that deserves support, rather than a disability that a child can be cured of. However, with a legitimate argument, a more radical section of the autistic community would say, 'Autism is not a disability, but a difference. We don't want treatment or cure, or to be labelled as having a disorder, but we do want societal understanding, acceptance and better work opportunities'.

What do you imagine happened to the first person diagnosed with autism by Kanner? His name is Donald Triplett, the 'first child of autism'. At the time of writing, he is still alive and recently had his 80th birthday party attended by 100 people. He has spent most of his life working as a bank teller, even continuing working after the official retirement age; a car driver, he played golf, mainly on his own, travelled the world, attended church and was be beloved in the community of Forest in Mississippi. Our understanding of autism has come a long way from the darker days of psychiatric diagnosis.

Cultural attitudes to autism and Asperger's have shifted over the two past decades. Donna Williams wrote in her autobiography *Somebody Somewhere* (1994) that being with other people with a similar condition at a conference gave her a sense of belonging, saying, 'together we felt like a lost tribe'. In 2004, two teenagers launched *Wrong Planet*, one of the first autistic spaces, on the World Wide Web. In the past few years, successful television programmes have popularised characters with Asperger's traits such as Sheldon in *The Big Bang Theory* (2007–2019) and the detective and central character, Saga Noren, in the Scandinavian detective series, *The Bridge* (2011–2018) and Dr Shaun Murphy in *The Good Doctor* (2017–20). The bestselling novel about a boy with Asperger's, *The Curious Incident of the Dog in the Night-time* (2003), is now a West End play, and *The Rosie Project* (2013) is a bestselling comedy novel about a man with Asperger's. *The Big Short* (2015) is a film about those financiers who predicted the financial crash of 2008, some of whom were definitely 'on the spectrum'. A friend of mine informed me that his 17-year-old daughter with Asperger's commented recently, 'Dad, I had a diagnosis of Asperger's before it became cool to have Asperger's'.

## Reasons, advantages and disadvantages for a diagnostic assessment

This greater awareness of autism has led to more adults seeking out a diagnosis later in life. The diagnostic service I work in started out with a trickle of referrals and there is now a flood with a ten-fold increase in referrals in the past 15 years. A diverse range of people come for assessment, from a professor at the local university who is married with children, to a single, unemployed man who has never had a relationship and has never worked. Some are impulsive and have attention deficit hyperactivity disorder characteristics, whereas others are careful and conscientious. Some struggle with language; others use it with ease and precision. The majority of people we assess have some mental health problems, particularly anxiety and depression. The people referred may have spent the majority of their lives wondering why they are different and never fit in, struggling with relationships and jobs, feeling anxious in social situations, blaming themselves for failures, but having never understood the underlying cause. Many people have adjusted to or can camouflage the characteristics; 'pretending to be normal' is a common survival strategy. In one recent study of women and girls, nearly every person interviewed wished they had known about their diagnosis earlier.

The main reasons that people come for an assessment are varied: (1) a third party prompts the referral: a partner, family member, clinician, doctor or someone in the criminal justice system. (2) The person might see something in the media, carry out an online questionnaire and recognise themselves, thinking 'Yes, that's me'. 'I just want to know; I just want peace of mind'. (3) They might have had a child or a relative diagnosed with autism and think, 'I see my five-year old as quite normal although he's been diagnosed with autism. I'm like that too'. (4) Sometimes, there is a crisis or tipping point at work, education or at home or a transition from a familiar structure such as leaving school. The person or their family might think, 'I need a diagnosis to get extra help at university' or 'I need a diagnosis to get social care'.

Seeking a diagnostic assessment is a big decision and could be a significant life event. There are advantages and disadvantages to take into account before reaching a decision to be assessed.

## Advantages

1 The diagnosis can provide a framework of understanding and an explanation of why a person thinks, feels and behaves as he or she does; it can help explain those difficulties and abilities to others. One person said, 'I blame myself less now, it's a kinder label than other psychiatric labels. It has helped me articulate things I didn't have the language to before'.

2 The diagnosis helps with accessing services and support, either at college or in the workplace, claiming benefit or support. The person has legal rights in terms of anti-discrimination under the Equality Act (2010).

3 Those with autism will find that they are no longer alone and can end that bewildering sense of isolation and loneliness. The person can become part of a whole community of like-minded people, if they so choose.

4 Gaining understanding of the positive aspects of being on the autism spectrum means understanding strengths as well as weaknesses. This may help with making decisions about work and direction in life.

5 The diagnosis might be more helpful to the person's family, friends and those around them in improving relationships, which in the past might have been characterised by misunderstanding and confusion. For example, Debbie came along for a diagnostic assessment with her daughter, Sally, and after a thorough assessment was duly given the

diagnosis of having autism. She commented, 'It doesn't make a great deal of difference to me', but Sally insightfully commented to her mother: 'The diagnosis is more for us, for me and my sister because now we will know how to deal with you and we can be more understanding. It's also for my husband who just thinks that you are arrogant and lazy – the diagnosis will help the family to understand you better'.

## Disadvantages

1 There might be a fear of exposure, vulnerability and rejection, especially if a person has spent all of their life creating a persona or mask of normality, hiding their real self. To expose their real self is a significant psychological step which involves some degree of loss, grieving and adjustment.

2 Younger people in particular do not want to be considered different and might be reluctant to accept a diagnosis. The diagnostic assessment has to be handled with care, at the right time, and the person has to be ready for it; otherwise, they are likely to feel stigmatised.

3 Relationships can change. People might view the person differently, making unhelpful assumptions. In marriage and families, feelings might change and in the work place, there may be discrimination, and the individual may find it more difficult to get a promotion or feel scrutinised.

## Not needing a diagnosis

Many people who might be somewhere on the autism spectrum never receive a diagnosis. There is no clear dividing line between people with autistic traits, or so-called eccentrics, geeks and boffins and people diagnosed with autism. Attwood (1998) describes this well: 'It is a seamless continuum that dissolves into the extreme end of the normal range ... there are people who have a "ghosting" or "shadow" of the condition' (p145). At their best level, they might be considered eccentric or unusual: they might be mathematical geniuses, computer whiz kids or artists. At worst, they might be people who are isolated, function poorly and might be considered to be lost souls, who slip into the psychiatric services. An important factor to take into account is the 'impact' of the symptoms on the person's life – on their education, work, relationships and mental health.

In my personal life, I regularly come into contact with neighbours, friends or acquaintances, who have autistic traits, which do not have a major negative impact on their lives and they do not seek a diagnosis. It is possible that for some people, a change of circumstances might create difficulties where they don't cope and having a diagnosis might actually help. I have a neighbour who collects old motor scooters and has an extensive knowledge of technical detail relating to engines, cars and computers. When we have a conversation, he will launch into a topic with a lot of technical detail and I will have no idea or interest in what he is talking about, but he will seem quite oblivious to my lack of interest. I also have a social worker friend who mentioned that he thought his younger sister was 'on the spectrum'. She had always lived at home with their parents, always carried out the same job in a library, always had the same sandwiches for lunch, never had a boyfriend or many friends and had little understanding of the complexities of social relationships, but she had an encyclopaedic knowledge of film, visiting the cinema twice a week on her own. Another friend has a son, who as a child, was suspected as having Asperger's but who never received a formal diagnosis. He was very rigid in his behaviour, insisting on having his food separated on a plate rather than mixed up, and at school got into fights with the school bullies because he felt that what they were doing was wrong. He had certain sensory sensitivities: hated loud noises, the sound of a vacuum cleaner and smell of lilies. Now in his 20s, he has adapted over the years; his social skills are better, although he still finds 'small talk' difficult, but does not see the benefit of having a label. A colleague commented about her ex-husband, who is a chief motor racing engineer, 'Gerry is definitely on the spectrum'. Amateur diagnosis of autism has become something of a trend, which hopefully doesn't trivialise the condition. However, I am sure we all know somebody who we might think is 'on the spectrum', and many of us recognise autistic traits in ourselves.

## Improving over time – growing out of a diagnosis?

As we grow up, we all develop skills and learn ways to compensate for our weaknesses. This is true of people with autism, who may develop, change and grow out of some of their autistic traits. A research study by Seltzer et al (2003) assessed 405 individuals who had met the diagnostic criteria for autism as children and found that only 55% met the criteria when re-examined as an adult. Another study by Howlin et al (2004) reported that 90% of people with autism show an improvement in autistic traits over the course of a lifetime and only 2% get worse. She identified a decrease in problem repetitive ritualistic behaviour and an improvement in reciprocal social responses. Individuals may still have symptoms, but they slip below the criteria for a diagnosis, because there is no significant impact on broader aspects of life.

On the subject of change and diagnosis, two people described different experiences in our clinic: one man said, 'I have socially re-engineered myself. I have had life coaching, training in non-verbal communication, social skills, speech therapy, public speaking, psychological therapy etc. I am now different to what I was, but it's all just a veneer; scratch the surface and I am still the same'. On the contrary, Jamie was 19 years old and wanted to join the army. He said, 'I can't get into the army with a diagnosis of Asperger's which

I have had since I was six years old. I think I've grown out of it. I want you to remove my diagnosis. My eye contact is better. I'm better at small talk, I'm not so obsessed by things and I'm less rigid'. Jamie had indeed made progress with social skills, scoring just below the diagnostic criteria and left the assessment a happy man heading for a career in the army. Liane Holliday Willey, the author of the bestselling book *Pretending to Be Normal* (1999, p133), said,

> Most of my Aspergic traits continue to fade away but some don't, they hang in there tenaciously cropping up to trip me over … Some-one called it Residual Asperger's. I have improved, my eye contact is better, but eye contact still makes me nervous. Small talk is do-able but in truth it bores me to pieces and makes me anxious. I can deal with change pretty well, but I prefer no change.

## Autism: a lens or mirror to view our own humanity

Hopefully, this book will paint a picture of autistic people as being 'different', not 'defective'. The progress of autism rights movement has been compared with other civil rights movements, the most common comparison being the LGBTQ community. Homosexuality was once a diagnostic psychiatric condition in the DSM (only removed in 1973), associated with treatments and cures. The emergence of the disability rights movement opposes the idea of autism as 'a medical condition to be cured' and sees it rather as a 'difference to be embraced'. Press coverage of autism has shifted from 'cause and cure' to 'acceptance and accommodation' as society has become much more accepting of diversity.

Many of the traits of autism tail off into personality characteristics found in the general population which many people can identify with. Understanding these traits can help us to learn more about ourselves, like looking into a mirror or through a lens, allowing us to see ourselves more honestly, and raising questions about our own human nature. It is possible to get a rough idea of where we are with respect to the autism spectrum by considering the following simple questions.

- Do you feel more comfortable alone than with groups of people?

- Do you enjoy chit-chat or small talk, just for its own sake?

- Are you a person who likes detail, needs to understand and collects information?

- Do you feel more comfortable expressing your thoughts rather than feelings?

- Do you like a settled routine and predictability or change and 'variety being the spice of life'?

- Do you hold very strong views and opinions about what is right and wrong or do you usually see the middle ground?

- Are you very sensitive to certain sensory experiences, feeling overwhelmed at times?

I enjoy working with autistic individuals because they are often refreshingly different, straightforward and painfully honest – with little or no social pretension. They often see the world and think differently in a creative, fresh, unconventional and imaginative way – having thoughts that most of us take for granted. They are often vulnerable, struggling awkwardly to understand and negotiate the nuances of the social and emotional world we live in. Autistic people are in some ways 'non-conformists', the ultimate 'anarchists'. They often don't obey the conventions, rules and norms concerned with celebrity, materialism and money, preferring comfort over fashion, work over play, hobbies over socialising, and thoughts over emotions. They often do their own thing and pursue their interests with a passion.

Adults on the spectrum have usually had a challenging time, and have the emotional scars that have resulted from struggling, surviving bullying and teasing and feeling isolated, marginalised and different. Working with autistic people teaches tolerance and understanding, acceptance and celebration of difference, diversity and compassion, indeed I have learnt greater acceptance of my own quirks and traits. It is about understanding human nature, both the head and the heart. It is about recognising that things don't always have to be perfect. Generally, autistic people do not rejoice over others' misfortunes. Life need not be about greed, lust, gossip, competition, trying to be 'top dog' or trying to get one over another person. If everyone sticks to the rules, there is enough for everyone without competing or getting the better of someone. An ideal life is about having a routine, doing work, having a task to perform, information to organise, someone to love, one or two friends and a limited amount of socialising. This book is based on the knowledge I have gained from working with this diverse population of individuals, from both their perspective and my perspective. It is my hope that it will lead to an improved understanding for both autistic people and those who work within the area.

# CHAPTER 2

# Theories and facts about autism

## What we know

Autism is a highly complex neurodevelopmental condition. Understanding of the condition has developed and changed significantly over the past 70 years, but its causes are still poorly understood. There is not one single theory of autism, but many different theories which together contribute to our understanding. This chapter will consider two key areas of theory and research. First, theories that look at the mind of people with autism; how information is processed, thinking and behaviour. Second, theories that focus on the biological level; looking at genetics, hormones and the make-up and connectivity of the brain. Let's start with a few basic facts about autism:

- Autism is a neurodevelopmental biogenetic condition, which means it is something a person is born with.

- Autism is not caused by bad parenting; it is definitely not the parents' fault. Theories in the 1950s and 1960s which used terms such as 'refrigerator mother' to suggest inadequate parenting were damaging, misguided, misleading and wrong.

- Autism is a lifelong condition. Autistic people may change, develop new skills or learn to mask traits associated with the condition, but talking about a 'cure' in a medical sense is not helpful.

- Autism has strong genetic links and runs in families, but there is consensus that there is no one single genetic difference. We do not know which particular genes are involved.

- Autism is best thought of as an umbrella term, which describes a range of different people, all with relatively similar behaviours.

- Autism is a spectrum condition. Like all people, autistic people have certain difficulties, to a greater or less extent, but being autistic will affect them in different ways. All autistic people are different.

- There is no link between the onset of autism and vaccination.

- Autism is more common in males than females. However, it is suggested that females are often not diagnosed because they learn to 'camouflage' their condition.

- Research indicates that autistic brains are wired differently; their neural connectivity affects the way information is processed.

- Almost eight in every ten autistic adults experience mental ill health, which is significantly higher than average.

## Theory of mind

Perhaps the most popular theory associated with autism is the theory of mind (ToM). This refers to a person's ability to recognise and understand the mental state of oneself and others – a form of imaginative mental activity that lets us perceive and interpret human behaviour in terms of intentions (e.g. feelings, desires, beliefs, reasons, purposes and goals). This is the ability to intuitively track what another person knows and thinks during personal interaction and then use that information to understand and monitor our own responses. Colloquially understood as the ability to 'put yourself in somebody else's shoes' or take a perspective other than your own is sometimes referred to as 'mentalising'.

ToM exists on a continuum, in some people it is more developed than in others. Autistic people have a relative weakness, as do people with schizophrenia, ADHD, various forms of brain injury and those who have poor early emotional attachments. A number of areas of the brain are linked with ToM, perhaps most significantly the medial prefrontal cortex (mPFC) which is located in the middle of the forehead, above the line of the eyebrows.

Good ToM, or the ability to 'read' others, correlates with more advanced social or people skills. Without a good ToM, life can be unpredictable and scary; misunderstandings and puzzlements may lead to conflict and distress as feelings and thoughts about others are unrecognised.

For most autistic people, ToM is not completely absent, but it is often acquired gradually and can lie dormant or be less extensively used. Interestingly, if an autistic person is asked, 'What do you think they are thinking?', they are likely to answer reasonably well. It is almost as if the autistic person needs external cues or prompting to discern, or 'hack out', the mental state of others; it does not happen as intuitively, naturally or spontaneously as it might in others.

Research suggests that most neurotypical (non-autistic) children gradually develop ToM, but for children on the autism spectrum, there appears to be a time delay and poor subsequent development. At 14 months, a child with autism has poor joint attention for carrying out tasks such as pointing and following another person's gaze. For example, if a person points their finger at something, the autistic child may look at the person's finger, rather than what they are pointing at – failing to read the intention of the person pointing. At 24 months, an autistic child may struggle to engage in pretend play. At 4 years, an autistic child struggles on tests that check whether they have developed the ability to take another person's point of view or perspective. At the age of 9, children with autism tend to perform badly in a test called the Faux Pas test that is failing to recognise what might hurt another person's feelings. Recently, in a study of young children, a selection of animated films and cartoons were shown and the children were asked what happened next. The autistic children could describe the physical aspects of the story, but were poor at describing the intentions or mental states of the characters.

## Weak central coherence

The weak central coherence theory suggests that autistic people are remarkably good at attending to detail, but appear to have considerable difficulty perceiving and understanding the 'larger whole', the 'overall picture' or the 'gist'. The autistic person's brain focuses on the detail first, tends to think in parts and does not fully connect all pieces of information in to a larger pattern of behaviour or thought – 'failing to weave together information to extract meaning'. When studying at school, the autistic person might learn vast amounts of information but struggle to connect, interpret, integrate and organise that information into an academic essay. The essay might be grammatically perfect and full of information, but poorly organised and fail to specifically answer the question. It's as if the person is looking at the world through a rolled-up piece of paper or a pipe and can attend to things in detail but is unable to 'see the wood for the trees'. An autistic person can get 'stuck in a groove', being unable to change, multitask or make new plans. This is sometimes referred to as 'bottom-up' processing, where the person starts with the details rather than the 'whole'. In comparison, non-autistic 'top-down' processing people have a tendency and drive to draw information together, 'to create an overall picture' and see 'the big picture' rather than the details.

In some circumstances, being able to ignore the bigger picture and focus on the details is an advantage; think for example of careers in maths, coding, programming, copy-editing, engineering and accountancy. However, in ordinary day-to-day life, being detail focused can be a disadvantage; one lady remembered her art teacher commenting on her painting saying, 'I don't want to see every blade of grass, I want to see a picture of a garden'.

Weak central coherence theory hypothesises that, as a result of detail overload (both from the social environment and sensory environment), a person will try to respond through control and order; to systematise, break things down into categories, create structures, routines and rituals, so that the world becomes orderly and more predictable. A sense of sameness is generated which feels safer and more comfortable.

## Monotropism and executive functioning

The core theory of monotropism, put forward by the autistic academic, Murray (2005), is that autistic people have a single channel of attention; they are in an attention tunnel where unanticipated changes are abrupt, uncomfortable and experienced as a disconnection. This explains why autistic people are often good at intense special interests or hyper focusing, but weak at processing multiple channels of input. For example, some autistic people find the combination of spoken word, body language and eye contact challenging, being unable to keep up with group conversation or the back and forth of neurotypical conversation. Monotropism also explains why autistic people are very literal in understanding communication; the monotropic mind is expecting one thing and is not primed for hidden meaning, metaphors, indirect language, sarcasm or the decoding of social implications. In fact, autism in young children is occasionally mistaken for deafness as the child's attention is focussed on one thing and might not register unwelcome interruptions.

There are similarities between the idea of 'monotropism', and the notion of poor executive functioning, a 'catch-all phrase' to describe difficulty with flexible thinking, multitasking, organising, planning and dividing attention. The theory of 'weak executive functioning' will be covered in more depth in the chapter on cognition (Chapter 5 page 65). However, in essence, it suggests that the frontal lobes of the brain, the executive, act like the conductor of an orchestra, integrating, engaging and disengaging different parts of the orchestra at will. The conductor may wave his baton and the violins join in, another movement of the baton and the woodwind section is hushed. However, in those with autism, the 'executive' or conductor is not as efficient. The shift mechanism is 'sticky', a little rigid, not as smoothly oiled; individual sections of the orchestra might play brilliantly but the overall sound is not as melodic or harmonious as intended.

## Empathising and systematising and the extreme male brain theory

Professor Baron-Cohen (2008) suggests that the two defining characteristics of autism are the skills of 'empathising' and 'systematising'; these are positioned in opposition – the more empathy you have, the less systematising you have. Empathising is the ability to recognise another person's state of mind and to respond with an appropriate emotion. It involves understanding the emotional and social world; being interested in others and sensitive to their needs and feelings, recognising emotion and distress and acting compassionately. In contrast, systematising is the drive to analyse or build a system that follows acknowledged rules. A high systematiser has a drive to analyse, spot patterns, construct systems and recognise the rules that govern those systems in order to predict how the system will behave. Systematisers are people who ask questions, particularly the question 'why', and who want to know how things work. Systematisers collect information; they might be interested in mechanical, numerical, language or any other system. Systematisers are 'researchers' in the broadest sense, preferring predictability and repeatable patterns, resisting change.

Generally, males score higher on systematising than females. Similarly, people with autism tend to score higher at systematising and lower on empathising. Baron-Cohen has likened this theory to the concept of the 'extreme male brain' – the title of his book. The second part of Baron-Cohen's theory is that there are clear sex differences between male and female brains. This is linked to prenatal levels of sex hormones, such as testosterone and oestrogen in the amniotic fluid, present in the mother's womb before the child is born. The higher the level of testosterone, the more the brain tends towards that of being a 'systematiser', or a classic male brain (liking to analyse and understand rules). Conversely, the lower the level of testosterone, the more the brain tends towards being a good empathiser, a more classically female brain (having better social skills, more empathy and a keener understanding of the emotional and social world).

Baron-Cohen's theory is supported by research into babies' early reactions; sex differences are present from the first day of life as girls are more likely to look at faces and boys more likely to look at mechanical mobiles. Furthermore, in the very early months, before the effect of socialisation, boys tend to prefer and are drawn to play with toy vehicles such as cars and trains, or construction toys like Lego, whereas girls tend to prefer to play with dolls. Higher foetal testosterone levels in childhood from 12, 24, 48 and 96 months is consistently correlated with measures such as poor eye contact, poor social skills, poorer ability to read emotion, lower empathy, higher systematising and other autistic traits.

However, Baron-Cohen's theory has been open to criticism and misinterpretation. First, Baron-Cohen is not saying that autistic people lack empathy. Empathy has, at least, two parts: cognitive empathy (being able to recognise what someone else is thinking or feeling) and affective empathy (having an appropriate emotional response to what someone is thinking or feeling). The evidence suggests that it is only the first aspect of empathy (cognitive empathy) with which autistic people struggle. Autistic people are not uncaring or cruel but may be confused by other people or be unable to identify another person's emotions. They may miss the cues in someone's facial expression or vocal intonation and may have trouble identifying with others (putting themselves in someone else's shoes). When the autistic person does notice somebody else's suffering, they usually find it upsetting and are as emotionally moved to want to help as anybody else – often more. A second potential misconception of Baron-Cohen's theory centres on gender; he is not saying that autistic people are hyper-male in general, or in terms of other typical sex differences. People with autism tend not to be extremely aggressive, but rather tend to be gentle individuals. Baron-Cohen's research is still in its infancy, but offers sound explanations.

## Special focused interests and routines

Imagine how chaotic and confusing life must be for the autistic child: with problems understanding the social and interpersonal world, a brain that focuses on details rather than wholes, challenges with language and the intense bombardment of sensory stimulation as the brain fails to filter out unwanted sensory information. How to cope with all this this confusion? One theory is that the young autistic person tries to create routine, rituals, repetition, structure and sameness to promote calmness and stability. Special focused interests emerge out of this need to make order out of chaos and the need to achieve coherence.

Once the interest is developed, it can be enormously soothing, relaxing and calming because it is regular, ordered and secure. The interest offers a sense of coherence, predictability and certainty in life. One man said: 'The world is chaotic, frightening and disorganised, but organising something like my rock collection helps me shake off that feeling of chaos that comes from living in such a frightening disorganised world'. Often the more stressed the person's life, the more pronounced the interest becomes. The focused interest is also a source of pleasure often greater than socialising. It allows a development of expertise, boosts self-esteem, provides something to talk about, provides an identity and sometimes can create friendships. One autistic man defined a friend as 'someone with similar interests'. It also offers the opportunity to escape into an alternative world.

These special interests are a form of systematising, often involving an accumulation and categorisation of knowledge and facts about a particular specific, narrow, obsessive area, understanding the rules of how things work, spotting patterns. Tom commented, 'Facts are important to me because they make me feel secure and comfortable in what is otherwise a very unstable world'. These interests, according to the diagnostic textbooks, are an 'encompassing preoccupation or restricted patterns of interest that are abnormal in either intensity or focus'. The interest might be a mechanical system (an engine or computer game), a natural system (the weather or animals), a numerical system (timetables, calendars, finance or coding/programming), a collectable system (rocks, cards and badges), a language system (learning a language). Unusual or special interests can develop very early in life – as young as 2 years. Sometimes it might commence with spinning the wheels of a toy car, lining up toys or collecting coins or pencils or Thomas the Tank Engine. David became an avid collector, and as his collection increased, he developed a cataloguing system almost like a library. He said:

> When I was younger, I used to collect comics and keep them in neat piles on the shelves in my bedroom and I'd read them over and over. On one occasion I noticed that a story line had been repeated two years after it first appeared and so I wrote to the comic. They replied and apologized, but then they did the same thing again a year later.

Autistic girls seem to have less obvious special interests than boys, perhaps because they are more interested in trying to be social. Girl's interests often include animals, particularly horses, or people, pop stars or bands, drawing or fantasy books like Harry Potter. Indeed Harry Potter was a bit of an outcast who turns into a triumphant hero, a figure with magical power – a figure people with autism can identify with easily. Girls seem more interested in learning about social relationships often tending to watch soap operas on TV or read fiction, partly as a way of learning about social relationships. For some girls, their special interest might include 'themselves', or trying to understand the psychology of human behaviour. See Table 2.1 below for a list of common special interest.

*Table 2.1* Common special focussed interests

| | |
|---|---|
| Transport/mechanical | Trains, planes, ships, cars, tractors, buses, Thomas the Tank Engine, washing machines, lawnmowers, maps, road systems, metal detecting, dustbin lorries, clocks |
| Science | Mathematics, coding/programming, engineering, fossils, global warming, geology, astronomy, timetables, weather, lexicology, technical side of film making, outer space |
| Pets/animals | Horses, dogs, dinosaurs, ants, insects, reptiles, quails, tropical fish, unicorns, owls, sharks |
| Strategic games | Computer games, online role-playing games, Minecraft |
| Creative/artistic interests | Drawing, music, art, writing, language, film making, fantasy world |
| Comics/cartoons | Anime, Manga, Marvel and DC comics |
| Films/books/TV | *Harry Potter, Lord of the Rings, Star Wars, Star Trek, Red Dwarf, Dr Who,* fantasy, UFOs, science fiction, true crime, Disney, Cult TV, SpongeBob |
| Collections | Lego, Pokémon cards, badges, sparkly things, matchbox cars, shiny things, bottles, rocks, My Little Pony, books, coins, stamps |
| Martial arts/sports | Taekwondo, Tai chi, Formula1, running, cycling, archery, chess, cricket, football, bell ringing, Pilates, bowls |
| History | First World War, Second World War, Vikings, Egyptians, conspiracy theory, Etymology (history of words), migration patterns |
| People | Pop stars, bands, actors, Sherlock Holmes, James Bond, Bertie Wooster, politicians |
| Self | Psychology, how humans work, myself, human behaviour, Philosophy |
| Less common interests | Cars made by the Rootes Motor Group, Mississippi Hill Country Blues, Mark 111 Cortina, Eurovision song contest |

The capacity to talk endlessly about a special interest can be a real strain for the rest of the family. The recollection of an elder sister to her autistic brother is typical: 'For years all my brother would talk about at the dinner table was bionicles (a type of Lego). I used to feel so angry I would sometimes shout at him. He couldn't conceive that anybody would want to talk about anything else. He has still got them lined up in his room 15 years later'. Autistic people often describe the overwhelming desire to talk about the subject whether or not anybody was interested and often in a monologue. The brother commented, 'I don't care whether they are interested or bored. I wanted to talk about it. It was like a spring within me that had to get out'.

## Compensatory strategies for being different

Attwood (2007) suggests that there are four main ways a young child copes with feeling different from other children; these can mask a diagnosis of autism. Attwood's theory, which is partly based on clinical observation, suggests that in order to survive, the autistic child consciously or unconsciously might adopt one, or more, of these strategies. The strategy chosen will depend on the child's personality, family, circumstances and experiences.

*Strategy 1: self-blame and depression*: those children who tend to internalise thoughts and feelings might become self-critical, blame themselves and become increasingly socially withdrawn. The child might desperately want to have friends but lacks the necessary social skills and recognises this as a failing. Low mood can lead to avoidance and a lack of energy which has an adverse effect on sleep and eating. Unfortunately, this appears to be the most common strategy.

*Strategy 2: escape into imagination*: some children escape into an alternative, internal world of imagination and fantasy, perhaps even creating imaginary friends. One client, Jessica, said: 'I didn't have any real friends and wanted to keep away from people, aside from my family. I preferred the company of my imaginary friend Sarah and her brother James'. Escape can also lead to an interest in other worlds, such as science fiction and fantasy, or possibly a passion for astronomy or geography, or another special interest. However, if that fantasy world becomes too extreme and the person becomes too detached from reality, they might be suspected of developing delusions.

*Strategy 3: imitation*: a constructive compensatory strategy is to watch, observe, learn and imitate other children or characters in books, films or TV, thereby camouflaging underlying autistic traits. Some autistic children become remarkably good actors, perfecting the ability to mimic and copy other people. However, whilst this strategy brings a veneer of social success, the person may still feel different and conscious that they are 'pretending'. In fact, some people become so accomplished at this pretence that they then have difficulty convincing others that they have real problems with social understanding and empathy. Females seem to use this imitation and camouflaging strategy more than males.

*Strategy 4: denial and arrogance*: children may overcompensate for feeling inadequate and ashamed in social situations by denying that there is a problem and pointing the finger of blame outwards. They see themselves as 'above the rules' and have difficulty admitting to being wrong or making a mistake, often arguing their case very skilfully. These children would not want to be referred for a diagnostic assessment and would likely find it difficult to accept that they have autism. In social situations, they can become dominating and controlling as a way of masking their own social insecurities.

## The 'female presentation' and 'camouflaging'

Over the last decade, interest in the 'female presentation of autism' has increased. Underpinning this idea is the assumption that females, either with or without autism, are superficially innately more sociable than males, which affects how autism manifests itself. The phrase, 'the invisible end of the spectrum' has been coined because girls often 'fly under the radar' or are better at 'camouflaging' their difficulties. Camouflaging or 'masking' is a form of 'impression management' where behaviour which occurs in front of others is, consciously or unconsciously, manipulated in order to make a better impression. One client said, 'I hide behind what I want people to see. I present a different identity to the world; covering up those parts of myself I'm not happy with'. It could be argued that autistic girls develop less severe, more subtle, softer-edged symptoms than boys because their social and communication skills and non-verbal behaviour is better; they also have less obvious restricted repetitive behaviours. Typically, women and girls are diagnosed later in life than boys (1.5 years later in children) and are less likely to be referred for a diagnostic assessment than boys. Autistic females are also more likely to be 'hiding' under other psychiatric diagnosis such as borderline personality disorder, anxiety, depression or an eating disorder such as anorexia.

There are a number of differences between the presentation of autism in males and females, with girls having the following characteristics:

- Stronger verbal and language abilities than boys.

- Better eye contact – girls seem to learn to do it, since it is does not come naturally, but report that it can be quite tiring.

- Greater awareness of the need for social interaction and an increased desire to interact with others.

- More imaginative; they might act out things they have seen during the day and can fantasise and escape into fiction and pretend play – imaginary friends are not uncommon.

- Less likely to use isolation as a coping strategy.

- Often good observers, being good at imitating, mimicking and emulating popular peers.

- Often have one or two good friendships and tend to be 'looked after' or protected in their peer group.

- Often perceived as, 'just being shy' rather than a 'loner'.

- May read fiction books and watch soap operas as a source of information about the social and emotional world.

- May be non-reciprocal, with a prepared script and overly controlled when playing with other children.

- Intense special interests; tend to be focused on people and animals (e.g. soap operas, celebrities, pop music, horses, drawing, fashion, pets and literature) rather than objects/things. Sometimes the special interest might be 'themselves' or the psychology of human behaviour.

- May have a tendency to be perfectionistic, very determined and controlling.

- Less likely to develop conduct problems than boys.

- Motor co-ordination problems are less conspicuous in the playground.

- Report more sensory issues than boys. Often dislike uncomfortable clothes because of sensory issues, around touch and texture, choosing comfort over fashion.

- Often 'get on' better with boys than girls. In groups of girls, the dynamics might be more nuanced, 'bitchy' and complex.

- Often good academically, well behaved and good at following the rules. They may even be 'top of the class', so will not alert the attention of teachers.

- Show fewer outward repetitive routinised behaviours, although may internalise them.

Case study: Louise

I realised I was different when I went to primary school. I would talk about things I was interested in, like cars, opera and Lego, but that was not what everybody else seemed interested in – there was a mismatch. I was always more comfortable in the company of adults and boys, although I did have one friend. I was bullied, but adapted to fit in. I learned from an early age about eye contact, and if someone makes a joke you are supposed to laugh. I copied gestures and imitated the popular girls – working out the social rules. I learned to be feminine, although I didn't really like it. When I got home I was exhausted. I spent my teens and early 20s trying to 'fit in'. Since getting a diagnosis aged 27, I've decided to drop the compensation, the camouflage, and the mask and just be me. When I tell people I'm on the spectrum the most common response is, 'You'd never know'. I think I've done such a good job of pretending that people often don't really believe me.

Perhaps the most extreme case of camouflaging I have seen was a 20-year-old linguistics student who came to our clinic recently. She asked, 'How do you want me to be, my normal self or my pretend self? I'm very good at pretending, I'm very clever'. We encouraged her to be her, 'normal self' and she proceeded to speak in a childlike, high pitched, slightly jerky voice, displaying poor eye contact and ill-directed facial expression. She evidently ticked all the boxes for a diagnosis of autism but left us questioning – 'Why hadn't her diagnosis of autism been picked up before?' And, 'How has she survived on her university course?' At the end of the assessment, we enquired as to what her 'pretend self' was like and she gave us a 2-minute 'performance', directing a conversation to her older sister who had accompanied her. She transformed into an unrecognisable figure; her voice was louder, deeper and more fluent; she used appropriate eye contact and gestures; she was confident and outgoing, mimicking the accents of her friend, who was not present and being quite entertaining. However, at the end of the session, she acknowledged that being her pretend self was very tiring and stressful.

It is important for those diagnosing autism not to focus solely on the surface behaviours but to ask probing questions and get underneath the camouflage. Unfortunately, the tools used to diagnose autism are probably biased towards the stereotypical male presentation. Therefore the clinician needs to use their 'clinical brain' and judgement rather than slavishly depending on inadequate assessment tools.

## Autism runs in families – the strong genetic link and other factors

There is no single genetic test or biomarker for autism and no single gene associated with the condition. Genetic research has identified over 100 genes harbouring mutations linked to the condition, but there is a frustratingly low rate of definite results. This might be because autism is such a heterogeneous diverse condition.

Recently, a number of large studies have confirmed that autism is a highly heritable condition, with approximately 80% heritability. This means that 80% of the influence on whether a person will be autistic is due to their inherited genes. Studies of twins have shown that if one monozygotic (identical derived from one ovum) twin is diagnosed as being on the autism spectrum, the likelihood that the other twin will get a diagnosis is 80%. Furthermore, one in five infants who have an older sibling with autism will also receive a diagnosis.

A further factor which increases the likelihood of developing autism is the age of the father; being born to a father over the age of 40 increases the probability of the child being autistic by six times, compared to having a father under 30. This is due to an increase in the level of mutations in a father's sperm after the age of 40. There is not thought to be an increased probability if the mother is aged over 40 (King et al, 2008). However, having an 'intelligent dad', whose IQ is over 111, is thought to increase a child's risk of autism by 32% (Gardner et al, 2020). A further strand of research indicates that 10% of extremely premature babies test positive for autism (Kolevzon et al, 2007). This is thought to be due to the babies' brains being exposed to many stressors during a very critical stage of development. Bacterial or viral infections in the mother during pregnancy have also been found to slightly increase the risk of autism in the offspring.

Volkmar's (1998) research reported that 46% of first-degree relatives (parents) of children diagnosed with an autistic spectrum condition shared similar autistic traits. Relatives often exhibited subclinical or autistic personality traits rather than a clinical disorder. This theory was developed by Baron-Cohen who identified that having a parent who worked in a so called STEM profession (science, technology, engineering and mathematics; all professions that require high-level systemising skills) increased the likelihood of familial autism.

Autism also appears to be linked with a number of unusual, rather diverse, physical conditions which include the following:

**Gastrointestinal dysfunction** – 80% of autistic people have gastrointestinal dysfunction, particularly children. Altered bacterial gut microbiology, endocrine and nutritional problems have been identified.

**Sleep problems** – These are twice as common amongst children with autism as they are amongst non-autistic children – 80% of autistic preschoolers have disrupted sleep.

**Hypermobility and Ehlers–Danlos syndrome** – These genetic connective tissue disorders, often called joint hypermobility or joint laxity, co-occur statistically more frequently in those with autism.

**Tuberous sclerosis** – A genetic condition caused by the mutation of one or two genes causing benign tumours and lesions to form in many different organs of the body. Between 25 and 44% of people with this condition have autism.

**Deafness** – Between 2 and 4% of children who are deaf are also autistic.

**Polycystic ovary syndrome (PCOS)** – This occurs in about one in ten autistic females and is thought to be associated with irregular menstrual cycles and the presence of high levels of androgens and testosterone. Mothers who have PCOS have twice the probability of having a child with autism.

## Autism prevalence rates

The prevalence rates of autism have changed quite dramatically over the past few decades. Around 40 years ago, it was thought that autism was rare, and the incidence was about 1 in 2500. Whereas today's incidence rates are estimated to be about 1 in 100 (Baird et al, 2006). In the United States, a study by the Centre for Disease Control and Prevention found that prevalence rates could be as high as 1 in 68 in 2014, rising to 1 in 54 in 2016 (CDCP, 2020). A recent study in Northern Ireland suggested 1 in 25 schoolchildren were diagnosed (DoH-ni.gov.uk 2020).

This increase in the prevalence of autism may be due to better recognition and understanding, but is there another explanation? The term 'associative mating' addresses the phenomenon that people who carry a risk gene for autism are more likely to meet and mate with others who carry similar risk genes. Putting the two risk genes together might produce a child with diagnosable autism; even if both parents only exhibited shadow traits of the condition. An article in *Wired* magazine (December 2001) noted the higher incidence of autism in places like Silicon Valley in California. This is an area where people with high systematising skills or attention to detail come together to work as IT specialists, programmers, coders and engineers. The article highlighted that whilst the incidence of autism in the general population was approximately 1%, in areas like Silicon Valley, it might be as high as 10%. Roelfsema et al (2012) showed that the Dutch city of Eindhoven, known as having a high density of science, techology and engineering workers, had over twice the prevalence of school children diagnosed with autism, compared with two other Dutch cities of similar size.

## The autistic brain – connectivity and wiring

Modern neuroscience has generated substantial evidence to suggest atypical development and difference in the autistic brain's structure and functioning. Our understanding of autism has moved from it being 'all in the mind' to being 'all in the brain' – from psychiatry to neurology. However, probably because the autistic community is so diverse, and the brain is so complex, there has been no definitive identification of any 'biological marker' or 'autistic part' of the brain; such a discovery would be like a key opening the door to an understanding of autism. However, let's examine the theory that autistic brains are 'wired' differently.

*Increased brain growth when young and poor 'synaptic pruning'*: research has identified that there is an unusual pattern of brain growth in the first 4 years in certain areas and that autistic brains are bigger and heavier.

The normal course of events, in the neurotypical brain, is that within years 2–4, there is a process called 'synaptic pruning' or culling. Brain neurons and synapses (connections) are initially overconnected to their neighbours, and as the brain develops, a process occurs where irrelevant connections are culled in order to increase the efficiency of neural connections – a little like pruning a rose bush. This does not seem to happen so efficiently in the autistic brain, leading to some areas being over connected and some being under-connected. However, this early growth spurt doesn't last long and by adolescence there is an accelerated rate of decline in size; by the age of 30, the autistic brain is the same volume as the non-autistic brain. Scientists are not sure exactly why this happens, but it is thought that there might be age-specific changes in gene expression, molecular, synaptic and circuit abnormalities.

*Over and under neural-connectivity*: researchers have looked at neural connectivity in the autistic brain and found that communication and the speed of processing information between different areas of the brain may be different. There is evidence that autistic brains have an excess of relatively short neuronal fibres – surface white matter which links areas that are close together – producing what is called, 'local over connectivity'. These short fibres (like short cables) can often imply that the person becomes very good at details. Conversely, those with relatively fewer longer fibres in the deeper white matter (or long distance cables) connecting distant parts of the brain are often poorer at perceiving an overall picture. This means that the different brain regions are less connected; regions are not talking to each other, or are 'out of synch'. The amount of information that goes from the executive or frontal lobes (where concepts are formed, plans are made and the overall picture is perceived) to the more distant detail-orientated areas at the back of the brain is relatively low. This fits in with the theory that autistic people are poorer at 'top-down' thinking and tend to be 'bottom-up' thinkers, starting with the details and then slowly building a picture. Imagine, for example, the effect of one auditory or visual cortical neuron being over-connected to lots of others – any stimulus or sensory input would be amplified like sound coming out of a massive pair of speakers. This sensory amplification and reduced ability to filter out unwanted sensory information is one explanation of the sensory sensitivities that people with autism experience.

*When your brain won't hang up*: recent research from the University of Utah (King et al, 2018) reported that symptoms of autism, such as difficulty shifting attention between thoughts or conversations, may result from sustained connections between different regions of the brain being slower to fade out when there is a required shift. Brain connections fade out more quickly for people without autism, whereas autistic people remain synchronised for up to 20 seconds longer. The research team described this scenario as being like having a telephone that won't hang up. The research also found that the more severe the autism, the longer the 'duration of synchronicity' or length of time before the connection disconnected.

## The autistic brain – structural differences

In 2011, a magnetic resonance imaging (MRI) study from the University of Louisville in the United States compared a group of autistic people with non-autistic people and measured their corpus callosum, the band of thick fibre (like a bridge), that connects the right and left hemispheres. They found that *sections of the corpus callosum were smaller* or differently shaped in the brain structure of most of the autistic group (see Figure 2.2). Within the corpus callosum, axon diameter and number were reduced which effected the velocity and volume of signal transmission. The researchers could distinguish between the groups on the basis of the corpus callosum length with a level of accuracy of around 82–94%. But accuracy rates at that level are not quite high enough for researchers to say they have discovered a 'marker' for autism. However, a smaller corpus callosum could explain limited connectivity among brain regions and help explain why autistic people have difficulty integrating complex ideas.

A second area of research has shown that autistic people have a *smaller, less connected cerebellum,* the walnut-like lump at the back of the brain that sits underneath the two hemispheres, behind the brain stem and is sometimes called the 'little brain' (see Figure 2.1). Its main role was initially thought to be smoothing out movement, small motor coordination, balance and dexterity, but recently it has been linked with social cognition, or

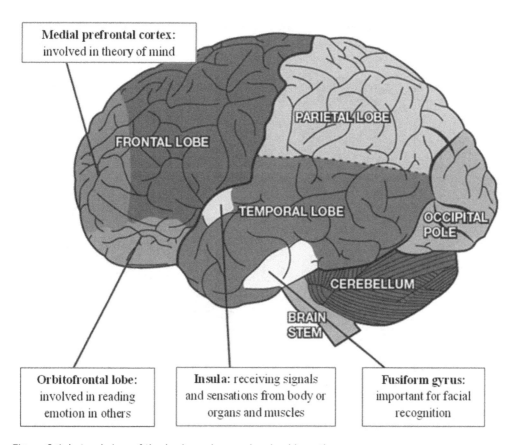

*Figure 2.1* Lateral view of the brain and areas involved in autism

building internal models of social behaviour. A damaged or smaller cerebellum may explain why people with autism can have poor coordination, tending to be clumsy, both physically and socially. The cerebellum in autistic people has a reduced number of purkinje cells – the cells involved with motor coordination.

A third area of note has been the *different activity levels in the amygdala*. The amygdala is the almond-shaped structure buried deep in the brain in each hemisphere, which plays a significant role in generating and regulating emotional responses such as fear and desire – it is the brain's emotional hub. It is often thought of as the body's alarm system, the primitive brain, which scans the environment for danger. We know from functional MRI (fMRI) studies that, depending on the particular task, the amygdala in those with autism can be significantly underactive or overactive.

*The social brain circuit is less connected*: when autistic people are engaged in tasks involving ToM (thinking about other people's thoughts, feelings, intentions or emotions), a network of brain regions, known as the 'social brain', can be less active than in the neurotypical brain on fMRI scans. Like lights on a Christmas tree, if there are poor connections and one of these regions of the brain doesn't work, the whole network suffers. The main regions involved in this circuit include *the mPFC* – this area is in the middle of the frontal lobes and is involved in the skills which compare one person's perspective to another person's, aiding understanding of thoughts and feelings. The *right temporal parietal junction* is involved in processing other people's actions, body perception, eye gaze etc. and helps us to judge another person's intentions and beliefs. The *right fusiform area* shows

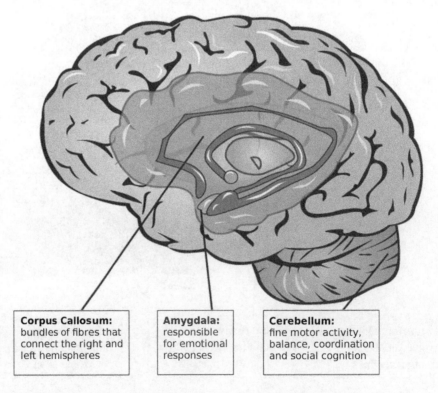

**Corpus Callosum:** bundles of fibres that connect the right and left hemispheres

**Amygdala:** responsible for emotional responses

**Cerebellum:** fine motor activity, balance, coordination and social cognition

*Figure 2.2* Medial view of the brain and areas associated with autism

abnormal activity levels in autistic individuals when processing faces. The *anterior insula* – thought to be the part of the brain involved in 'interoception' or the awareness and appraisal of our own bodily state, physiological condition, emotions, sensations and feelings, including pain – is believed to be less active and less connected in autistic people.

*Famous brains that are different: Albert Einstein and Temple Grandin:* individuals on the autistic spectrum may share some similar traits with each other, but it remains a very diverse diagnostic group. However, looking at specific individuals' brains can be very revealing; for example, Temple Grandin's and Albert Einstein's brains are particularly unusual. Temple Grandin, possibly one of the most famous autistic people in the world, an author and designer of humane cattle-handling facilities, has been involved in many studies of brain-imaging and has an intimate understanding of how her brain is different. She discovered that her brain is not symmetrical and is about 15% larger than the control subjects. Her cerebellum is 20% smaller than the average and, as this area deals with motor coordination, it would explain why her sense of balance and hand–eye coordination is poor. Within the brain, there are open spaces called ventricles, and the chamber or ventricle on the left-hand side of Temple Grandin's brain was 57% longer than the corresponding one on the right; her left ventricle is so long that it extends into her parietal cortex. A neuroimaging study also revealed that the white fibre tracts that snake through her brain from the frontal areas to the areas at the back of the brain that deal with spatial and visual memory (occipital) were overconnected. In her words:

> I must have an internet trunk line, a direct line into the visual cortex to explain my visual memory. I thought I was being metaphorical but I realise at this point that the description was a close approximation of what was actually going on inside my head. My brain isn't broken; it just didn't grow properly. Hence I see the small detail before the big picture.

There has been much speculation about the brain of Albert Einstein, who was considered by many to have had autism and had arguably one of the most famous human brains. A rather ethically questionable but strange story explains that the doctor who carried out Einstein's autopsy removed his brain from his skull unbeknown to his family and stored it in two large jars in his office. Later, with the advent of more sophisticated technology, it was analysed and found to be smaller than the average brain; weighing 1230 g rather than the average 1400 g – refuting the argument that the cleverer you are the bigger the brain. It was also found that the parietal lobes were unusually large, being 15% wider than average brains. The left parietal lobe had an abundance of glial cells (non-neuronal cells), significantly outnumbering neurons by 10–50 to 1. As the parietal lobes are involved in visual and spatial computations, mathematical thought and the imagery of movement, the extra brain material in this area could explain Einstein's spatial and mathematical prowess; it is said that he developed his theory of relativity by creating images and pictures of people on a moving train. Einstein is also known to have had delayed language skill; so his brain was likely to be weak on language and words but strong at visual and spatial tasks, which include mathematics.

> Thoughts do not come in any verbal formulation. I rarely think in words at all. A thought comes and I try and explain it in words afterwards. Words and language do not seem to play any part in my thought process.

Research on the autistic brain is fascinating but we are still left with the fundamental 'chicken and egg' question of, which comes first? Are people autistic because their brains are different or is a person's brain different because they are autistic? Is there something else – a protein, a mixture of genes, prenatal sex hormones, a different endocrine system – causing that difference? There is obviously a need for further research, but that research is hampered by the fact that autism is such a heterogeneous diverse condition. There is also a moral dimension: what if a cause for autism was found, would we want to intervene, reduce neurodiversity or not? I personally think the world is a richer and more interesting place with greater diversity - let's celebrate our differences.

# The diagnostic assessment

## The diagnostic assessment – a jigsaw

Greater recognition of autism in adults has led to an increasing demand for diagnostic assessments. As yet there are no simple biological markers such as a blood test or brain scan to identify autism, so a diagnostic assessment is required. Assessment is a lengthy process, often 3–4 hours or more, and involves an interview with the client, observation of behaviour, set tasks, questionnaires and review of information from other relevant sources. It is recommended that an assessment is multidisciplinary; in our service, a clinical psychologist and speech and language therapist work together to assess if the diagnostic criteria are met. Where possible, it is recommended to involve a client's family member or partner in the process to provide collateral information, especially about the early years of the client (neurodevelopmental history). In many respects, the diagnostic assessment interview is 'detective work' on the part of the clinician trying to piece together the evidence. Attwood (2007, p50) uses the metaphor of a jigsaw puzzle to explain the process.

> I explain to the client and family the concept of a 100-piece jigsaw puzzle. Some pieces of the puzzle (or characteristics of Asperger's syndrome) are essential: the corner pieces and the edge pieces. When more than 80 pieces are connected the puzzle is solved and the diagnosis confirmed. None of the characteristics are unique to Asperger's syndrome and a typical child and adult may have perhaps 10 to 20 pieces or characteristics. The person referred to a diagnostic assessment may have more pieces than occur in the typical population, but sometimes not enough, or the key or corner pieces, to complete the puzzle and receive a diagnosis of Asperger's syndrome.

The diagnostic process is not a precise science; if we accept the theory that autistic traits lie on a spectrum or continuum, it is inherently problematic. Attwood (2007, p52) explains that the decision can be subjective.

> The final decision on where you draw the artificial line, namely whether a person has a diagnosis of Asperger's syndrome is a subjective decision made by the clinician ... based on the clinician's clinical experience, the current diagnostic criteria and the effects of the unusual profile of abilities on the person's quality of life.

However, the value of the diagnosis should not be underestimated. It is not just a label but a passport or signpost for support, as well as a key to open the door to greater understanding.

## The diagnostic statistical manual (DSM-V)

In order to obtain a diagnosis, a medical classification system has to be employed, where often the language is unfortunately couched in terms of 'disorder' and 'deficit', rather than 'difference'. We try and strike a balance, accepting the need for a diagnostic framework, but trying to employ non-deficit language and emphasising strengths. There is no single definitive method that professionals use to make a diagnosis, but most follow the diagnostic criteria set out in either the DSM-V or the International Classification of Diseases (ICD-11). These comprehensive catalogues set out the prerequisites for diagnosis based on a number of criteria and symptom areas. Specifically, the DSM-V states that:

- The symptoms must be present in the developmental period, in the early years before the age of 8 years old; therefore, a thorough neurodevelopmental history is important.

- The symptoms must cause significant impairment or impact in social or occupational functioning or mental health.

- The range of symptoms cannot be explained by other causes such as intellectual disability or other medical or genetic conditions.

The range of symptoms is broken down into two main groups or domains which some people have been likened to a constellation (see Fig 3.1). To obtain a diagnosis, a client has to meet the criteria for all three categories in Domain 1 and at least two out of the four in Domain 2. Importantly, even if the traits were apparent in childhood but are not present in adulthood, the criteria can still be met.

*Domain 1: Persistent deficit in social communication and social interaction across multiple contexts.* There must be evidence of difficulties in all three of the following categories:

(a) *Deficits in social–emotional reciprocity.* For example, this may range between an abnormal social approach and failure of normal back-and-forth conversation to reduced sharing of interests or emotions and failure to initiate or respond to social interactions.

(b) *Deficits in non-verbal communication behaviours used for social interaction.* These may include poorly integrated verbal and non-verbal communication, abnormalities in eye contact, use of gestures, lack of facial expressions and body language and deficits in understanding the non-verbal communication of others.

(c) *Deficits in developing, maintaining and understanding relationships.* For example, this may range between difficulties adjusting behaviour to suit various social contexts to difficulties sharing imaginative play or in making friends and an absence of interest in peers.

*Domain 2: Restricted, repetitive patterns of behaviour, interest or activities.* There must be the presence of difficulties in at least two of the following categories:

(a) *Stereotypical or repetitive motor movements, use of objects or speech,* for example, simple motor stereotypes, lining up toys or flipping objects, echolalia (repeating or echoing phrases) or idiosyncratic phrases.

(b) *Insistence on sameness, inflexible adherence to routines or ritualised patterns of verbal or non-verbal behaviour,* for example, extreme distress at small changes, difficulty with transitions, rigid thinking patterns, greeting rituals, needing to take the same route or eat the same food every day.

(c) *Highly restricted, fixated interests that are abnormal in intensity or focus,* for example, strong attachment or preoccupation with

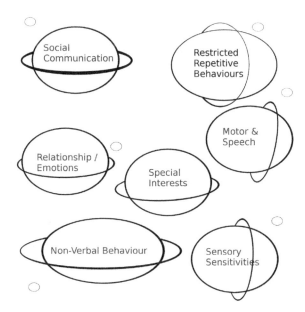

Figure 3.1 The constellation of autism's clusters of symptoms

unusual objects, excessively circumscribed or perseverative (repetitive) interests.

(d) *Hyper- or hypo-reactivity to sensory input or unusual interests in sensory aspects or the environment,* for example, apparent indifference to pain or temperature, adverse response to specific sounds or textures, excessive smelling or touching of objects, visual fascination with lights or movement.

## The clinical interview and the client's neurodevelopmental history

The process of assessment usually starts with the client and a relative being sent out screening questionnaires; these are scored and provide useful background information. Following this, during the first part of the assessment, a standardised semi-structured assessment tool, which includes a mixture of live conversation and structured tasks, called the 'Autism Diagnostic Observation Schedule' (ADOS) Module 4 (2016), can be used to explore the client's communication skills. However, remember this tool doesn't always pick up either the 'female presentation' or the presentation of older adults who have learned and developed social communication skills over the years. A short break may need to be taken to allow the clinicians to score the ADOS-4 and confer.

The second part of the assessment is a detailed fact-finding clinical interview which explores neurodevelopmental history and other criteria related to the DSM-V categories. Consideration of the client's family history, education, employment, relationships, mental health, reason for referral and current functioning will be discussed. Once enough information has been gleaned, the clinicians may have a second short break to discuss and complete the scoring grid (see the end of the chapter). A decision regarding diagnosis is usually fed back to the client and their family member or partner at the end of the session.

### Neurodevelopmental history

This is an in-depth examination, looking for clues of autism during the first 8–10 years of life. It is ideally based on an interview (or questionnaire) with parents or a third party such as an elder sibling or relative. This information forms the cornerstone of the neurodevelopmental exploration and enhances the reliability and validity of the assessment. The following selected questions are based on The Relatives' Questionnaire (from the Autism Research Centre, derived/taken from the Childhood Asperger Syndrome Test [2002]). The client is sent the questionnaire beforehand, with the request for a parent or relative to complete it, then it is used in the assessment as an item for discussion.

1 Were there any complications with the birth or pregnancy?

2 Did s/he meet typical milestones for sitting up and walking at the appropriate age?

3 Did s/he have normal eye contact or was there some gaze avoidance?

4 Did s/he have sensory issues around being touched? Did s/he like to be picked up, cuddled and enjoy physical affection?

5 Was s/he speaking or 'putting words together' by 2 years or was there a delay and unusual use of language?

6 Did s/he play any pretend, imaginative or role play, make-believe games?

7 Was there an early liking of repetitive routines, rituals and inflexibility? E.g. was s/he a 'picky eater', or did s/he like to wear particular clothes or have strong attachments to particular objects?

8 Did s/he have good attention to detail, noticing things that others missed?

9 Did s/he have conversations just to be sociable (chit-chat or small talk), or was their conversation restricted to getting their needs met or talking about special interests?

10 Did s/he join in playing games with others and find it easy to interact with other children?

11 Did s/he come up spontaneously for a chat?

12 Did they have friends or play with a group of peers outside school?

13 Was it important for her/him to fit in with peers and did s/he care about how s/he was perceived by peers?

14 Did s/he tend to take things literally?

15 Did s/he get invited to other children's parties and if so, did s/he enjoy them?

16 Did s/he have poor motor coordination or clumsiness – did s/he enjoy sports?

17 Was s/he sensitive to noises, lights, textures, smells, tastes or show unusual responses to temperature or pain?

18 Did s/he like to do things over and over in the same way?

19 Could s/he keep a two-way conversation going, taking turns appropriately?

20 Did s/he have the same interests as his/her peers?

21 Did s/he have an interest that took up so much time that s/he did little else?

22 Did s/he bring you things s/he wanted to show you?

23 Did s/he enjoy joking around?

24 Did s/he have difficulties understanding the rules of polite behaviour?

25 Did s/he have an unusual memory for details?

26 Was her/his voice unusual in any way?

27 Were people important to her/him?

28 Did s/he say things that were tactless and socially inappropriate?

29 Did s/he have any unusual or repetitive movements, such as rocking, flapping, walking on toes, or hand and finger mannerisms?

30 Was his/her conversation difficult to follow or make sense of?

31 Did s/he often steer conversations to talk about a special interest?

32 Did s/he have odd or unusual phrases or make-up words?

33 Has s/he ever had difficulty reading or had a diagnosis of dyslexia, dyspraxia or had hearing difficulties?

34 Did s/he ever refer to themselves in the third person e.g. 'Oliver wants to…', rather than, 'I want to…'

35 Did you, teachers or health professionals ever express any concerns over her/him?

36 Any other comments…

Sometimes, the neurodevelopmental history points very directly towards a diagnosis. In the following example, a mother who accompanied her 36-year-old daughter to the assessment describes her daughter's childhood.

> She was a quiet baby. If you picked her up, she would cry. She was happier if you laid her down and wrapped her up tightly in her blanket. She was a little late in walking, but once she did, she just stood up and started walking. There wasn't much in between such as crawling. The same with talking and potty training; once she got the idea, she was absolutely perfect. Her first words weren't mummy or daddy as you would expect but, "Thomas the blue engine." When she started speaking, she had a very strange tone and was very formal for a small child, a bit like an adult talking. She has grown out of that now. She was a happy child but very much in her own little world. If I left her, she would just be happy to sit on a blanket playing with her toy cars or train. She didn't obviously see the

consequences of something – if she was hot, she didn't immediately
see the sense in taking her cardigan off or if she was hungry didn't
obviously see the sense of putting food in her mouth. She would get
really upset – beside herself – with the sound of the vacuum cleaner,
or when her younger brother came along and he started crying. I
was a little scared of her, because if something upset her, the reaction was always extreme – so for a lot of the time I felt that I was
walking on eggshells. Things had to be a particular way or it would
create a problem. She had to have all her buttons done up and her
shoelaces fastened very, very tightly; otherwise there would be a
tantrum. Once when she went to a party she hadn't got the idea that
you are supposed to smile and talk to people and she just sat in a
chair in the corner on her own. At school she just focused on her
work. I remember she was made "date monitor" at primary school
and the teacher said, 'She is the most reliable date monitor I've ever
had in 20 years of being a teacher.' She actually got on much better
with the adults and teachers than the other children.

Other parental testimonies are less insightful. One parent said, 'I didn't
notice anything; it all seemed quite normal. He was quiet, polite and
happy to be on his own. He had a few unusual habits, but was the perfect
child'. Such a response may be for a variety of reasons: the child might
have been very self-contained and compliant and slipped under the radar
of detection due to camouflaging; perhaps, there were other more bois-
terous siblings or peers distracting attention away; perhaps, the child
escaped into their own internal world; perhaps, the parents themselves
might have had some autistic traits and didn't notice their offspring's
difficulties.

For most people on the autistic spectrum, life before getting a diagnosis is
a struggle; people often comment, 'I always knew I was different but I didn't
know why'. Many have had a bewildering childhood and don't understand
the logical social norms, fashions and unwritten rules of social behaviour:
'When I went to nursery school it was odd because I didn't know what
I was supposed to do. I just didn't get being a kid. I never understood the
rules'. Isolation is a real problem: 'I'd be the one standing on my own in the
playground'. Many autistic people are teased and bullied at school which
results in developing low self-esteem: 'I was terrified for most of the time at
school; I didn't know what was going to happen next'. Many children are
tricked and manipulated because of their naïveté about social relationships
and a lack of ability to read others' intentions. One way to survive involves
careful imitation and modelling, watching how other people manage. A man
recalled an event from his childhood which was particularly painful: 'I saw
children running about in the playground hitting each other – they must
have been playing tag – and I thought, 'That's how you make friends.' So,
I started running around randomly hitting people and it was a disaster –
I got told off by the teacher'.

## DSM-V criteria: Domain 1: Persistent deficit in social communication and social interaction across multiple contexts

When assessing on the basis of the DSM-V criteria, the clinicians will have to make a judgement based on their observations of the client's behaviour. The DSM-V instructs that (1) behavioural difficulties have to be clearly atypical and occur across multiple contexts (2) some behaviours may appear to satisfy multiple DSM-V criteria, but it is the responsibility of the clinician to decide where the behaviour is best represented and not put one behaviour in multiple criteria. For example, 'repetitively putting hands over ears' may satisfy criterion B1 because it is a repetitive motor movement but it may also be considered for criterion B4 because it represents an adverse sensitivity to sound. The following questions can either be used to ask the client or source of information directly or act as a prompt for the clinician to aid their decision-making. Bear in mind that the client may not have full insight into their own behaviour.

*Criterion A1: Difficulties with social initiation and responses*: This section involves assessing whether the client can have a back-and-forth reciprocal conversation, a verbal 'to-and-fro' dance about a topic that is not one of their special interests; carry out 'small talk' or 'chit-chat'. Is the person 'socially awkward, their conversation slightly 'out of sync'? Also, can the client report events in a coherent manner? Can they show interest in the assessor/clinician by, for example, asking questions? Can they share enjoyments, opinions and interests? This section is based on a combination of questions and observation.

1 *Do you struggle to have back-and-forth, turn-taking, reciprocal conversations?*
  (a) Are you good at taking turns in conversation? Can you build on comments that others make?

  (b) Do you have a tendency to 'talk over' or interrupt the other person?

  (c) Have you been told you frequently turn conversation back to yourself or your own topics of interest?

  (d) Is it possible that you tend to think more about what you want to say, rather than what the listener might want to talk about?

  (e) Do you have a tendency to get into one-sided conversations or monologues?

2 *Do you have difficulty with small talk or social chit-chat with others?*
  (a) Do you find that you don't enjoy small talk or social chit-chat?

  (b) Do you struggle to think of something to say to keep conversations going?

(c) Would you agree with this statement: 'I cannot see the point in superficial social chit-chat unless there is a clear discussion point, debate or activity'?

(d) Do you tend to initiate conversation only if there is a purpose or to get help?

(e) Do you sometimes cope by deliberately preparing a 'scripted' conversation?

(f) Do you have difficulty entering into a social group or initiating conversation?

3 *Would you say that you had limited interest in sharing your experiences, interests or achievements with others?*
   (a) Do you tend to share enjoyment, interests, news or achievements with other people, for example around the dinner table?

   (b) Would you say that you generally lack interest in the thoughts, experiences and opinions of others and tend not to ask questions in conversation?

   (c) Do you experience and show pleasure in social interactions?

   (d) Do you tend to get excited if somebody has good news?

4 *Have people said that they sometimes struggle to follow your train of thought clearly when you are reporting or explaining events? Similarly, do you sometimes struggle to follow others' conversations?*
   (a) Have people told you that you have a tendency to jump from topic to topic in conversation so they can't follow what you are talking about?

   (b) Do you have a tendency to focus too much on details, rather than the overall picture?

   (c) Do you have a tendency to struggle to get to the point and summarise information?

   (d) Do you have a tendency to ask for clarification in a conversation? E.g. saying, 'can you explain what you mean?' or saying, 'sorry, you've lost me', or, 'could you clarify please?'

---

### A1: Clients' examples of difficulties with social initiation and responses

1 My girlfriend says that I don't do the normal 'ping-pong' in a conversation, but instead give a monologue.

2 I have a strong desire to say what I want to say, irrespective of what the other person has said. If it's a subject I have genuine enthusiasm for, words flow out like a 'babbling brook'.

3 There is a bunch of magic rules to having a conversation that I don't know. For me, I just say what I mean and mean what I say.

4 I can't work out when it's my turn to talk and I can never think of what to say.

5 I can't keep track of conversations in a group situation – it moves too fast. I'll often say, 'Just go back to what you were saying about …'

6 I get really confused and frustrated if someone interrupts me when I'm talking about something I'm very interested in – I have to finish.

7 I interject or butt into conversations, sometimes with something unrelated.

8 I'm told that I talk at people, rather than with people – but I have to say what I think. My wife says, 'You're preaching again'.

9 I find it difficult to judge how much or how little people want to hear. People say to me, 'Too much information'.

10 I don't seem to be able to explain things succinctly or get to the point quickly. Instead, I go all round the houses. I can't summarise or précis.

11 My mind tends to jump around and I don't always explain to people where it's jumped to.

12 My friend said, 'You go too far', but I never know how far too far is.

13 I communicate with my parents on a need to know basis, or if there is a problem.

14 I've never celebrated any achievement; I just think, 'So what?'

15 My worst nightmare was getting an award at work for my database and having to go to a swanky dinner – I didn't want to talk to them.

16 I'm told I talk over people; I often mistime conversations, interrupt and when I do speak it's like an 'exorcism'.

17 Either I haven't said a word or I've said a thousand too many. I can't gauge what people want.

18 My wife says, 'Can I have the short version', otherwise I go on and on.

19 Sometimes when I start 'rabbiting' on about something, people say, 'It's like guesswork trying to work out what you mean'.

20 I can't see the point of small talk; it seems like a complete waste of time. I'd rather be discussing something important.

21 Going to the hairdresser and having to talk to him is more stressful than having three men with guns trying to kill me.

22 With small talk, I don't know what they want. I don't sense it.

23 I only speak when I need to speak; if there is a purpose or I want something.

24 Why would you talk about the weather when you already know what it's like?

25 I get bored with conversations that don't contain information.

26 I don't chat. On Monday morning at work, I say, 'Where is the work?'

27 I've learned a little script over the years and will say, 'How are you?' and make a comment about the weather.

28 I ask for clarification at least once in every conversation, saying, 'What do you mean?', or, 'Was that a joke?', or, 'Could you explain please?'

29 If somebody is talking, I am raring to go, desperate to find a gap and talk about what I want to talk about.

30 I tend to focus on my own thoughts rather than on what the listener might be thinking.

*Criterion A2: Difficulties with non-verbal communication*: Non-verbal behaviours are the tools we use to enhance and regulate social interaction and to recognise the communication signals the other person is giving off. The assessor/clinician is looking at both the client's expressive range of non-verbal behaviours (e.g. eye contact, facial expression, gestures, speech volume and intonation etc.) and their receptive ability to understand the non-verbal behaviour of others. Again, observation plays a large part in this section.

1 *Do you think that your range of non-verbal behaviours – such as eye contact, gestures, facial expression, speech intonation – are limited or unusual in any way?*

(a) Do you have difficulty or discomfort with eye contact during conversation?

(b) Do others comment that you use your hands to gesture too much, or not at all?

(c) Have you ever been told that your facial expressions are limited or inappropriate for the situation or do not match your feelings?

(d) Have you ever been told that your speech is flat and monotonous and doesn't vary with emotions?

(e) Have you ever been told that you have an unusual voice (e.g. too loud, soft, quick or 'jerky')?

(f) Have you ever been told that you are 'difficult to read' as you don't show emotion on your face?

2 *Do you struggle to read and interpret other people's non-verbal behaviour?*

(a) Do you sometimes struggle to recognise when someone is interested or bored with what you are saying?

(b) Do you have difficulty working out what someone is thinking or feeling just by looking at their face?

(c) Can you work out what people mean when they change their intonation pattern to indicate sarcasm?

(d) Do you have difficulty spotting if someone in a group is feeling awkward or uncomfortable?

(e) Do you have difficulty telling if someone is masking their emotions, or says one thing and means another?

(f) Do you have difficulty 'reading between the lines', identifying another person's intentions or recognising sarcasm?

---

### A2: Clients' examples of difficulty with non-verbal behaviour

1 My eye contact has improved over the years but I still find it uncomfortable, unnatural and too intrusive.

2 I look at the tip of their nose, forehead or mouth, anywhere but the eyes.

3 Do you want eye contact or a conversation? I can't do both. I find looking at someone's eyes very distracting. My best conversations are usually sitting alongside somebody whilst driving in a car.

4 I don't know how long to look. I end up staring at people.

5 I used to get teased at school and be called 'dead face', because my face doesn't have much expression.

6 I'm told I've got a 'dead-pan' expression and don't use many gestures or facial expressions when I'm talking.

7 I'm told my facial expression doesn't match my feelings. I might feel sad but someone will say, 'You look bored'.

8 I forget to pull the right facial expression, if I'm focussing on eye contact.

9 I've been told that I only use gestures when I'm angry and then I tend to point rather vigorously.

---

10  I can't talk without moving my hands. So, if I've got my hands in my pockets I've got nothing to say.

11  My wife says I speak too loudly and don't vary my volume in different situations.

12  I find it difficult to modulate my voice; people often accuse me of shouting.

13  I can only pick up extreme or obvious emotions. Someone is bored if they are yawning, looking away, trying to leave the room or looking at their phone. They are angry if they raise their voice and their face goes red. Sad if they start to cry. But it's the subtle in-between emotions I have difficulty with.

14  The book 'Body Language for Dummies' has helped me tell if someone is getting bored.

15  I find it difficult to work out people's intentions and read between the lines.

16  If I'm going to understand people they need to speak directly, clearly and specifically to me, rather than making inferences like raising their eyebrows or rolling their eyes.

17  I can't tell if I've upset Nicky until I see tears on her face.

18  I can't tell if someone is flirting with me.

19  I often say, as a check out statement, 'Am I missing something here?'

20  I say to my wife, 'I'm not a mind reader; you've got to tell me if you are upset or if you want me to do something. Be direct and specific; let's get rid of the mystery!'

*Criterion A3: Difficulty with relationships*: This section explores the client's ability to develop and maintain peer relationships and friendships appropriate to their age, and to be able to engage in and understand social situations. Potential obstacles are explored, such as lack of insight into what the ingredients are for a good friendship, the tendency to be too honest, blunt or direct, difficulties adjusting behaviour to suit the social context, lack of interest in others or need for social contact and lack of understanding of emotions of self or others (emotional intelligence).

1  *Do you have difficulty making and maintaining friendships?*
   (a) Do you find it difficult to make new friends?

   (b) Do you find it difficult to judge how another person is feeling about you, for example that they might want to be your friend?

   (c) Would you say that you find the unwritten rules of social behaviour a mystery?

(d) Do you wish that you had more friends but don't know how to make them?

(e) Do you prefer to have just one or two friends at a time?

(f) Do you find interacting with younger or older people easier than interacting with your peers?

2 *Do you enjoy joining in with social occasions or parties?*
(a) Do you tend to struggle with or avoid social occasions, such as parties or 'leaving dos'?

(b) Do you find it hard to know how to act in social situations?

(c) Do you prefer your own company and have a lower than average need for social interaction?

(d) If a friend calls at your house, without planning or warning, would they be welcomed spontaneously?

3 *Do you have a tendency to be very honest and straightforward, saying things without considering the emotional impact on the listener (making a faux pas)?*
(a) Have you been told that your comments are too direct, honest or blunt?

(b) Have you been accused of 'being rude' or offending others or making tactless comments even if you didn't mean to?

(c) Do you often clash with other people because of holding strong views and finding it difficult to compromise?

(d) Do you tend to overshare with friends and strangers?

4 *Do you have good insight into how relationships work and the emotional world?*
(a) Do you have difficulty recognising your own emotions and what triggers them? For example: first can you describe what things make you experience, or trigger the following emotions: second describe how you know that you are feeling that emotion, what is happening in your body, what sensation?

- Happy

- Afraid

- Anxious

- Angry

- Sad

(b) Would you struggle to identify things that you do that might annoy or irritate other people? Identify two things you do that might annoy others. Identify two things that others do that annoy you.

(c) Do you struggle to describe other people's personalities? Describe the personality of your father and mother.

(d) Have you ever found it hard to tell if someone is teasing, mocking or taking advantage of you?

(e) What does being a friend mean to you? How do you know somebody is your friend?

---

### A3: Clients' examples of difficulties regarding relationships

1 I find friendships too difficult, too effortful and tend not to bother with them.

2 I prefer to do things on my own rather than with others – I just don't have the need for social interaction.

3 I do not enjoy social occasions and tend to make excuses or avoid them. If I do go, I often feel exhausted or ill afterwards.

4 I can't see the point of going out for coffee and 'catching up' … what does it mean?

5 I had a friend come around to the house unexpectedly once and I didn't know what to do. My mother said, 'You were like a rabbit in the headlights'. He ended up playing with my brother.

6 I spend all my time in my room on my computer and don't have any real friends.

7 I have an absolute inability to lie, which overrides any sense of politeness. I wish I could keep my mouth shut and 'play the game', because I just end up upsetting people.

8 I'm better in social situations if there is a shared purpose, something to talk about, like going to my cycling or photography clubs.

9 I'm very territorial about my home. A few people are welcome by invitation only, but if people just appear at the door, I really don't like it.

10 I've had three main relationships with women in my life and they all say to me, 'You're a closed book; you don't give yourself away'. I've got no idea what they are talking about.

11 I'm too blunt and say things that upset people, but there is no malice aforethought … I don't mean to.

12 The rest of the world is so slimy, telling lies, bullshitting, not being straight forward. I tell the truth.

13 I would not be a good diplomat – wars would start.

14 I often offend people. Truth is one thing that people often don't like. I am 100% open and honest and can't lie or 'sweeten the pill', not even a 'little white lie', which upsets people.

15 Sometimes, I offend people by saying what I am thinking, even though I don't mean to.

16 I don't really understand political correctness. I'm always putting my foot in it. It just comes out of my mouth before the social filter kicks in.

17 When my sister was upset, I didn't know what to do. I just sat in silence and stared at the floor. I didn't know what to say. I thought, 'Shall I put my arm around her?' and then thought, 'How long is this going to go on for?'

18 I don't really understand how I'm feeling most of the time, so how can you expect me to understand how other people are feeling?

19 When I'm not physically present with my wife, whom I do love, I rarely think about her or miss her.

20 I don't think I have emotions. I mentally feel emotions.

21 If I get angry it's a flare-up, an outburst and then it's gone – there is no carry-over.

22 I was not very good at picking out if people were bullying or teasing me at school or whether they were really interested in me. It was all confusing.

23 My husband says I'm not empathic. The worst example was when he came and told me about his cancer scare and my initial reaction and comment was to say, 'What bank account does the child benefit go in?'

## DSM-V criteria: Domain 2: Restrictive, repetitive patterns of behaviour interests or activities

(Remember, difficulties need to be manifested in two out of four criteria, either at present or in the past)

*Criterion B1: Atypical patterns of movement and speech*: This category looks at repetitive patterns of movements (e.g. rocking or repetitive hand movements etc.), speech (e.g. pedantic, overly formal or echoed, repetition etc.) and use of objects (e.g. lining up objects or attraction to spinning objects etc.) These are 'things the person does because it makes them feel good'.

### B1: Atypical movement and speech
1 *Do you have any repetitive motor mannerisms (e.g. hand or finger flapping, rocking or twisting) either now or in the past?*

(a) Do you do any repetitive flapping (stimming) or flicking movements with hands or fingers or with objects?

(b) Do you or have you in the past ever repetitively rocked, skipped, spun, walked on toes, complex whole-body movements or repetitively jiggled your leg?

(c) Have you been told that you pull unusual facial expressions, grimaces, involuntary movements?

(d) Do you ever make repetitive vocalisation, such as humming or grunting sounds?

(e) Do you repetitively pick at your skin or scalp?

(f) Would you say that you had poor coordination, dexterity and sense of body in space? Were you poor at sports?

2 *Do you use objects in ways other than they were intended (e.g. twirling a piece of string, chewing an object, fiddling with an object)?*
   (a) Have you ever been absorbed by things that spin, such as a washing machine, a fan, or wheels?

   (b) Have you ever repetitively turned lights on and off, twirled a pen in your fingers, opened or closed doors or lined up toys or objects?

3 *Do you use language in an atypical way?*
   (a) Has anybody ever said to you that your use of language is formal or overly precise (as a child speaking like an adult or 'little professor')?

   (b) Would you say that you have a preference for exact use of words or precise information? E.g. will you give precise dates, such as 15 August 2019 rather than say 'last summer'.

   (c) Do you repeatedly use certain words or phrases?

   (d) Have you ever been described as pedantic, either giving too much or too little information?

   (e) Do you make up words, phrases, sometimes repeat or echo jingles or particular phrases in conversation?

   (f) Have you ever referred to yourself by your own name, or in the second person, rather than saying 'I'?

### B1: Clients' examples of atypical speech and motor mannerisms

1  As a child, I used to spend a lot of time spinning. Now I just do a slight rocking. It's comfortable and nice. I don't know I'm doing it until somebody points it out.

2  I make noises to myself like 'uurm ...', 'urm ...', a humming noise, like the noise of the car.

3  I'm always making noises, humming, tapping or singing, but it drives me mad if somebody else makes a noise.

4  I walked on tip toes when I was a child – people called me 'twinkle toes'.

5  If I get excited or stressed, I flap my hands – someone said it was called stimming.

6  I flick my nails together.

7  I have this thing where I twist my hair all the time or pick at my skin.

8  My leg shakes and I crack my knuckles when I feel anxious.

9  When I'm walking, my arms don't swing in time with my legs.

10  I arrange my fingertips so they are exactly lined up and also rotate my feet from the ankles.

11  I wear a soft, chewable necklace called 'chewellery', which I chew instead of chewing my hands or fingers.

12  I can't jog, I can only sprint – it's one pace, and the only way I can dance is to dance really quickly – I just seem to have one way of doing things.

13  I have been told that I'm clumsy and uncoordinated.

14  I'm always knocking things over; I can't catch or kick a ball to save my life and was always falling off my bike when I was a child. I never had a sense of natural grace; it was as if my brain and body were not connected properly.

15  I have never been good at team sports but liked solitary sports that required endurance like distance running and cycling.

16  When I was a child, I used to speak like an adult, like a 'little professor', and people would tease me by asking me questions and then laugh at me when I answered them. I couldn't really tell if they were teasing me or being serious.

17  There are certain favourite phrases I like using and sometimes people say I overuse them.

18  My parents say I sounded like a little grown-up when I was a child.

19 My girlfriend says that I speak too formally because I say things like, 'I recall', rather than 'I remember', or if she says, 'Do you want a cup of tea?' I say, 'No thank you, I don't want a cup of tea'.

20 I don't like it when people say my father is 'a postie', it's sloppy. I much prefer saying that my father works for the Royal Mail, or at the very least, 'My father is a postman'.

*B2: Routines, rituals, sameness, resistance to change in thinking and behaviour:* This section is examining inflexibility in both behaviour and thinking, which manifests in an adherence to specific routines, rituals and repetitions, with a desire for structure, order, predictability and sameness with a resistance to and distress with change. Thinking tends to be 'black and white', literal, with difficulty understanding irony, humour or implied meaning.

1 *Do you have a very strong adherence to specific routines or rituals, having to do things in a particular way?*
   (a) Do you have set day-to-day routines, with multiple-step sequences of behaviour (e.g. insistence on the same route, or food)?

   (b) Do you have routines that other people think are unusual?

   (c) Do you have to have things planned out in your head?

   (d) Do you collect things, categorise or arrange objects in a particular way (e.g. belongings etc.)?

   (e) Do you have rules that you like to follow and expect others to follow?

2 *Do you prefer to do things in the same way, over and over again, struggling with change?*
   (a) Do you like to settle into a regular routine and then see no need to change it?

   (b) Do you get very upset when the way you like to do things is suddenly changed?

   (c) Do you get very annoyed when possessions and belongings get moved or rearranged by others?

   (d) If there is an interruption, do you struggle to switch back quickly to whatever you were doing?

   (e) Do you have a tendency to watch films or a television programme over and over again?

3 *Would you say that you have a rather 'black and white', 'all or nothing', thinking style, where there is little room for 'the middle ground' or 'shades of grey'?*

(a) Do you have a tendency to think of issues as being black and white (e.g. politics or morality) rather than considering multiple perspectives in a flexible way?

(b) Do you have a strong sense of social justice, about what is 'right or wrong', with a refusal to compromise?

(c) Do you find it difficult seeing the other person's point of view in a discussion and find it difficult to change your opinion?

(d) Do you get frustrated if things are not clearly defined? When others say, for example, 'It depends', or 'How do you feel' or ask 'open ended questions', which seem vague?

(e) Do you find it difficult to do more than one thing at a time (multitasking)?

4 *Would you say that you have difficulty with imagination and tend to take things literally?*

(a) Would you struggle to make up a spontaneous imaginary story?

(b) Did you tend not to engage in make-believe, imaginative or pretend play as a child?

(c) Would you prefer reading (1) factual, technical, non-fiction or science fiction books as opposed to reading (2) fiction or novels about real life?

(d) Do you find it difficult recognising the implied or hidden meaning in speech (e.g. someone saying, 'You are the apple of my eye'), often missing the point, nuance or gist?

(e) Do you find it difficult recognising sarcasm, irony, jokes and certain types of humour?

---

**B2: Clients' examples of repetitive, routines, rituals, thinking and resistance to change**

1 My life is ruled by lists, sub-lists, goals and bullet points.

2 I prefer to do things over and over in the same way – it keeps me calm.

3 I need structure and plans and if somebody interrupts me, the whole day is ruined.

4 If I go into town, I need to know in what order we are going to go into shops and how long we are going to be there and when we are going into McDonald's. If the order goes wrong, I throw a massive tantrum.

---

5   I get extremely upset when the way I like to do things is suddenly changed.

6   I get upset if my mum moves anything in my bedroom.

7   I need to know what is coming next. Holidays have to be well planned – my route in the supermarket is planned. I don't like unexpected change to my routine.

8   In my head, I've decided what I'm going to do – I've made a plan, the pieces are all laid out – I don't like sudden changes which means reorganising the pieces.

9   I have all my CDs and DVDs organised in a particular way, all my clothes are colour and type coded – nothing is random.

10  I love playing the scales on my piano and like Mozart and Baroque music because it's neat, has a steady beat, phrasing with regular intervals so you know where you are. I don't like music by Wagner or Beethoven as it's more dramatic and all over the place.

11  When people say, 'We'll have to agree to disagree', it drives me absolutely mad, because it's either right or wrong, surely?

12  With me, it's either one or the other, there is no in-between.

13  The policy said, 'Leave to manager's discretion'. That is really annoying and too vague.

14  If I'm doing one thing, I'm doing one thing. I can't do two things at a time or be interrupted.

15  I don't like different foods touching on a plate. I keep them separate and eat them separately.

16  Everything to me is polar. I am the most polar man in the universe. In my head, everything is right or wrong. I never say, 'Oh, I'm not sure'.

17  I hate autumn when the leaves are half off the trees – I'd rather they were all off or all on as in winter or summer.

18  I couldn't play at having a tea party with a bear and a doll because in my mind that's just stupid.

19  My sister would play with dolls but to me they were just plastic things.

20  I can't imagine anything – it has to be right in front of me. In fact, the word imagination fills me with dread.

21  I loved Space and Technic Lego but couldn't build anything spontaneous like my brother. I'd have to follow the instructions. I couldn't make something from nothing. But give me instructions and I can produce something beautifully crafted.

22  At school, in a music lesson, we once did jazz improvisation and the teacher asked me to improvise 'Take the A Train'. I just

couldn't do it, yet I could play the clarinet fluently to Grade 8 standard. I was absolutely lost. It was so embarrassing. I just broke down.

23 In ballet, the teacher said, 'Do a 30-second improvised movement'. I couldn't think what to do and just rocked from foot to foot and everybody laughed.

24 I'd rather do a hundred sums than write a story. Making something up is very difficult for me.

25 I have never had any interest in things that were not real. Why would you read fiction when you could read something that was real and you could get something out of it?

26 A novel is not even a true story; why read something that is not real?

27 There is no such thing as 'a little white lie', it's either the truth or a lie.

28 I take things very literally; you have to say exactly what you mean – no inferences.

29 I don't get jokes, innuendo or sarcasm. I need people to talk directly and clearly and to say what they mean.

30 Someone said, 'He wears his heart on his sleeve'. I had no idea what he was talking about.

*Criterion B3: Intense or unusual interests*: This section is looking at whether the person might have special passionate interests that are all-encompassing or time-consuming, with a rather narrow range and very intense deep focus. A special interest is a form of systematising, collecting information and facts, understanding the rules of how things work, spotting patterns, distinguishing between types etc. With this systematising comes a special eye for detail and a perfectionistic need to get things just right.

1 *Do you have all-encompassing preoccupations or special interests that are unusual either in intensity or focus?*
  (a) Do you tend to get obsessed with certain topics that take over many aspects of your life?

  (b) Do you find yourself talking, thinking or reading about it, collecting information or items, or cataloguing aspects of that interest?

  (c) Do you frequently get so absorbed in one thing that you lose sight of other things?

  (d) Do you have interests that are very intense and narrow in focus, compared to the interests that others might have?

(e) Do you like to research and collect information about categories of things and have a large store of factual information (e.g. dates, models, types of cars, capital cities, types of birds, sports etc.)?

(f) Do you have a desire to understand how things work, often asking the question, 'Why?' repetitively, and wanting to research and drill down into topics?

2 *Do you have an 'eye for detail' or a persistent preoccupation with noticing parts of objects or systems?*

(a) Do you find that you tend to focus on the details rather than the overall idea?

(b) Do you have a passion for, or notice, or have a particularly good memory for car number plates, dates, numbers, passwords, telephone numbers, words or other strings of information?

(c) Do you tend to notice patterns, details and small changes that others do not?

(d) Do you have an unusual attachment to a particular object, which you like to have with you?

(e) If someone moved one of your possessions in your room, even slightly, would you notice?

3 *Do you consider yourself a perfectionist and have to get things 'just right'?*

(a) Do you have difficulty varying your own pace of work, or varying quality, or cutting corners when carrying out a task?

(b) Do you have difficulty prioritising, deciding what the most important aspect of a task is and what is least important?

(c) Do you have a strong need to complete or finish a task properly, before moving on?

---

### B3: Clients' examples of special interests

1 To me, my special interest is like a proper love affair. I love it. One of the reasons I married my husband was because he was also interested in Egyptology.

2 If I didn't have responsibilities, all I'd do all day is play on the computer and play with Lego. For a 36-year-old man, I like Lego too much. My wife bribes me to go shopping with her saying she'll buy me Lego.

3 I frequently get so strongly absorbed in one thing that I lose sight of other things.

4 If I get an interest in something, I have to collect information and research it to bits and completely understand it, and then I move on.

5 I've always loved maps and road systems. For my 16th birthday treat, my parents drove me around the M25.

6 I'm not very good at multitasking or standing back because I get sucked into details.

7 I will shop for an item by remembering the barcode.

8 When I was a child my family called me 'Charlotte Why', because I was always asking the question, 'Why?' – always wanting to understand things.

9 I am totally obsessed with the North American fur trade between 1860 and 1880.

10 I liked Thomas the Tank Engine because each train had its own colour, number and name; they all had set personalities that didn't alter and are quite predictable.

11 I have always been a collector. When I was young, I collected comics and kept them in neat piles, then it was badges, then Pokémon cards, now it's lawnmowers.

12 I've always been interested in military history.

13 When I was young, I became interested in fossils. Now I work in a museum and can't believe people are paying me for doing something I love.

14 For years all I would talk about at the dinner table was Pokémon or Harry Potter. It used to drive my sister mad.

15 Painting my models is so soothing and calming in times of stress. When I'm doing it, I never feel depressed – it's a natural antidepressant.

16 All the autistic people I know are researchers – we want to know and understand things. I find a hook and I drill down.

17 I could look at a document and scan it with my eyes. All the typos, spelling and punctuation mistakes jump out and I wouldn't be able to let them go.

18 At work they called me 'the error police' or 'the red line police' as I would notice errors on duty charts, or spelling mistakes would leap off the page. I always excel at writing down policies and procedural documents and believe in 'getting it right'.

19 I usually notice car number plates and other strings of information and can remember every phone number, password or door code I've known.

20 I know the bus timetables for the whole of Plymouth.

21  My art tutor said, 'I'm not interested in every blade of grass; I want a picture of a garden'.

22  As a child, I was always found with my nose in a book – usually about natural history or dinosaurs.

23  If I start something, I have to finish it and get it just right – there are no half-measures with me. I have to sort things out in my head, get them perfect, before I can say them.

24  I have seen *The Lord of the Rings* films over 30 times each. I like watching them because I know what's coming – I'm an expert!

*Criterion B4: Atypical sensory experiences*: This section examines how autistic people are often either hyper- or hypo-reactive or sensitive to sensory input, or certain aspects of the environment, whether it be to noise, light, touch, taste, smell, or temperature, pain, appetite or movement. Reactions are often extreme, as in strong aversion or attraction.

1  *Do you have a particular sensitivity to noise?*
(a)  Do you find certain loud noises unusually painful and distressing (e.g. alarm, hoover, siren, drill, a baby crying etc.)?

(b)  Do you often notice small sounds that others do not notice (e.g. ticking clock, people eating or people breathing)?

(c)  Do you have difficulty following conversations when there is a lot of background noise?

2  *Do you have a particular sensitivity to touch?*
(a)  Are you unusually sensitive to any light touch on your skin?

(b)  Do you cut the labels or tags out of your clothes?

(c)  Do you find that you are overly sensitive to certain textures (e.g. wool) and dress for comfort rather than fashion?

(d)  Do you like deep pressure such as tight hugs, tight body warmers or heavy blankets?

(e)  Do you only do handshakes if essential?

(f)  Do you find common self-care tasks like having a shower, haircut, cutting nails, brushing teeth etc. uncomfortable or painful?

(g)  Do you particularly like to touch certain textures or find them calming? E.g. a soft fidget toy or scarf?

3  *Do you have a particular sensitivity to light?*
(a)  Do you find a certain type of intensity of light, or bright lights, (such as neon lights, or bright sunlight) painful or hard to tolerate?

(b) Have you ever had a fascination with certain lights, shiny things or spinning objects?

4 *Do you have a particular sensitivity to taste?*
(a) Do you find it impossible to eat certain types of food because of the unpleasant taste or texture e.g. slimy food or crunchy food?

(b) Do you separate food on your plate or eat items individually rather than mixing and/or avoid putting sauces on food?

(c) Would you say that you have a restricted diet, or has anybody said that you are a fussy eater?

(d) Do you have a distinct preference for either very bland food or highly flavoured food?

5 *Do you have a particular sensitivity to certain smells?*
(a) Are you unusually sensitive to certain specific smells (e.g. perfume, aftershave, bleach), often to the point that if you can't escape them, you'll become physically ill?

(b) Are you strongly drawn to certain smells, textures or visual patterns?

6 *Do you have a particular sensitivity or insensitivity to temperature, pain, appetite or other bodily sensations?*
(a) Do you have an unusually high tolerance of pain?

(b) Are you unusually sensitive or insensitive to temperature?

(c) Are you good at noticing the early stages of bodily sensations such as, if you are beginning to feel hungry, thirsty or tired?

7 *Do you worry about sensory overload - being overwhelmed?*
(a) Do you sometimes feel so overwhelmed by your senses that you have to isolate and shutdown or run the risk of having a 'meltdown'?

---

**B4: Clients' examples of sensory sensitivities**

1 School was a sensory nightmare, with the noise of the bell ringing, the playground, the fluorescent lights, the smell of disinfectant and people bumping into me in the corridor.

2 I often notice small sounds when others do not.

3 I always cut the labels out of my clothes.

4 I can't stand the sound of a bell, hoover, alarm or hairdryer.

5 I can't stand the noise people make when they eat – I prefer to eat on my own.

6 I hate the sound of people breathing.

7 As a child, if I was given a doll, I didn't play with it but I liked to touch her hair. I touched her hair so much her head fell off and then I carried that around with me.

8 I really like the citrus smell of kitchen scourers and carry one around in my handbag and occasionally smell it during the day.

9 I always wear the same black soft cotton clothes – for me with clothes, it's always 'comfort over fashion'.

10 Wearing jeans feels like being encased in sandpaper.

11 I don't like being touched softly – it burns, it hurts like being cut by a razor. I'd rather be squeezed firmly.

12 When I feel overwhelmed by my senses, I have to isolate myself to shut them down.

13 Wool is the devil and I hate velvet!

14 When one of my senses goes, or gets overwhelmed, e.g. if the lights are too bright, all my senses go or get overwhelmed.

15 I wear sunglasses and earplugs to block out excessive light and sound.

16 I constantly notice and look at minute particles and pick up small pieces of fluff.

17 I can't wear perfume or stand the smell of aftershave; they give me a headache.

18 I find light fascinating.

19 Sometimes, touch is a problem because it's a massive distraction. If I'm at full mental capacity, I haven't got time to cope with it.

20 I can never tell whether I'm full or hungry and I never feel too hot or too cold.

21 I can easily recall the pitch of a tuning fork 5 minutes after it has sounded – I have perfect pitch.

22 I used to walk around constantly with my grandmother's silk scarves when I was a child. I loved the sensation. I called them my 'silkies'.

23 I shake a person's hand with gritted teeth.

24 I'm a very fussy eater and can't stand slimy food or (different) foods touching each other; I eat one food at a time and never put sauce on it.

25 Peas shouldn't touch ketchup – it's not allowed.

26 I don't notice if I'm getting hungry, then suddenly I'm starving.

27 I can't follow a conversation if there is a lot of background noise – if it's a radio, I turn it off.

28 I fell over in the playground once and only went to the hospital the next day because my parents insisted; my arm was broken. I didn't really notice the pain.

29 I really like deep pressure – such as a heavy blanket or my tight body warmer. They help me feel the edges of my body.

30 I don't feel fear like other people. My mum is always going on about being worried about me when I'm wandering around town late at night.

*Criterion C: Symptoms present from early childhood*: Is there definite evidence that the array of current traits has been present since early childhood (age 10 and younger)? Refer to neurodevelopmental history.

*Criterion D: Symptoms together limit and impair everyday functioning*: Does the impact of the range of traits significantly impair functioning in education, work, social life, relationships or mental health? Refer to personal history.

*DSM-V summary table*: Clinicians use Table 3.1 as a checklist to both direct search during the assessment and to clarify thinking and decision making at the end of the assessment.

*Table 3.1* DSM-V summary table

| DSM-V criteria | Evidence | | | |
|---|---|---|---|---|
| Criteria | None | Limited | Moderate | Significant |
| **Criteria A (all 3 required)** | | | | |
| **A1: Difficulties with social initiation and responses** | | | | |
| **A2: Difficulties with non-verbal communication** | | | | |
| **A3: Difficulties with relationships** | | | | |
| | | | | |
| **Criteria B (2 required either in past or present)** | | | | |
| **B1: Atypical movements and speech** | | | | |
| **B2: Rituals, routines and resistance to change** | | | | |
| **B3: Intense or unusual interests** | | | | |
| **B.4: Atypical sensory experiences** | | | | |
| | | | | |
| **Criterion C: Symptoms present from early childhood** | | | | |
| **Criterion D: Symptoms impact everyday functioning (work/study, social, family/relationships, mental health)** | | | | |
| **Third party verification** | | | | |

# Diagnosis – in my own words

## Telling the story

Each autistic person will have their own story. For many, a late diagnosis can be a turning point in their life as they continue on a journey of self-discovery and acceptance. In telling their story, they are able to make sense of their condition; to create an internal narrative or structure on which to build a new understanding of themselves; to realise, perhaps for the first time, that they are not alone and to learn from other people's stories of struggle and acceptance. In this chapter, nine autistic adults share their stories as they reflect on their journey of diagnosis.

Up until 1987, there were only three published autobiographies of people with autism. Publications on personal *growth* through *autobiographical reflection steadily grew in the 1990s*. Liane Holliday Willey's book, *Pretending to Be Normal* (1999), suggests that autistic traits continue to fade away, whereas Temple Grandin's book *Thinking in Pictures* (1995) puts forward the view, 'Autism is part of who I am. I am a condition of hope not a disorder'. Between 2003 and 2008, there were 30 more published, and since then there have been many more. The majority of these books celebrate the unique qualities of people on the autism spectrum and stress that although their path in life might be difficult, particularly before diagnosis, there are many positive aspects.

## Kate's story: 'Diagnosis stabilised my mental health'

Why am I different? Why can't I be like the others? Why am I always in trouble when I'm not being naughty? Why am I so useless? These were the questions that were a running commentary while I was young. I didn't understand how I could understand mathematical concepts so much earlier and quicker than others but couldn't figure out how to join in at playtimes. I was incredibly lucky that I was sent to a very small school and there wasn't any bullying. I would watch the groups playing or just stand on the edge, not joining in. I did have friends but I could only normally engage with one at a time and felt left out very quickly if there were more. I used to be sent on holiday with French families in summer and everyone used to think I was homesick, but I wasn't missing my parents. It took me a long time to figure out what was upsetting and challenging me – which was the change in routine, not knowing what we were doing and when.

These feelings carried on as an adult. I became very depressed as I couldn't figure out why I found life so difficult. I was labelled as spoilt, attention seeking or even having borderline personality disorder. I was frequently told that as I was highly intelligent, I didn't need to have angry outbursts, meltdowns or shutdowns. Often, I'd have meltdowns because I couldn't make anyone understand what I was feeling. How could I? I didn't know what it all meant or what I was actually feeling myself.

In early adulthood my life gradually came undone. I could not get out of the depression and thought it was better to die than to live like that. It was after a serious suicide attempt that I saw a psychologist who specialised in diagnosing adults with Asperger's syndrome. The Community Mental Health Team, whom I had been seeing, had had enough of me and had nothing left to offer and just saw me as a nuisance – they didn't think I had Asperger's.

I remember being able to talk to the psychologist – I'd found a YouTube clip of him so I knew what he looked like! I even managed to ignore his rather chaotic room (organised chaos, he told me!). The experience was interesting and actually quite enjoyable, and the ethos was that although I might think and behave differently from most people, that is all it was – different, not wrong. For the first time in a long time, I felt valued. It was so important to me that I could ask questions as we went along. At the end, he told me that I was definitely Asperger's. I felt I could breathe. With his explanation, how I felt all my life made sense. It gave me 'permission' to feel how I did, to find life as confusing as I did.

Afterwards when I told my parents, I remember them saying that they felt guilty as they'd believed I was just naughty and difficult. We had to draw a line – they couldn't have done anything different, because in those days people didn't know about Asperger's. They did what they thought was right at the time and let's face it, I am difficult, Asperger's or not!

The diagnosis has helped me in so many ways. With a diagnosis, medical professionals seem to listen when I explain why something is so hard. It has made me more aware of triggers, and I have accepted that I need to remove myself from situations that I know are difficult for me to handle. Most of the time I can tell myself that I am 'allowed' to feel like I am, but at other times, I still revert to the thought, 'I'm intelligent, why can't I change this?'.

I can honestly say that my diagnosis was the best thing that has happened. Whilst I still get frustrated that I can't deal with certain things, I am able to be kinder to myself, most of the time. I do not shy away from telling anyone who is involved in my life that I have Asperger's. The choir that I sing in accepts me as I am. I do not expect people to fully understand, but if they can give me space and some support, that's fine. What I would really like this world to know is that just because I am intelligent, it does not mean that I 'choose' to act the way I do when it is all too much and I am overwhelmed; too much noise, too much light, too much socialising! I have lived with my parents for the past few years and the diagnosis has certainly helped. My parents now realise that I am not necessarily unsociable but I need that down time when I come home from work. They also accept that I need routine and clear instructions. The anxiety, which we now realise, is more to do with the Asperger's than the depression, is more successfully managed by understanding the need for structures and warnings about change.

I believe that now I am getting the support I need due to my official diagnosis, and people are making adjustments. For those who believe diagnosing an adult serves no purpose, I totally disagree as I believe that it stabilised my mental health and saved my life.

## Joanna's story: 'Drafting a map to chart my course'

When I was 10 years old, we were driving through Colorado on a family holiday when my dad spotted a snowy hillside that was just perfect for sledging. We didn't have any sledges with us, so my dad fashioned some by unclipping the lids of our suitcases. On my first run, I realised why suitcase lids were not sold as sledges – they have no steering – and I hit an enormous bank of snow. Tumbling headfirst, I entered the snowdrift and was buried six feet deep. Inside, all was white. I was stunned and had lost all points of reference; I couldn't tell which way was up. Even today it feels as though I was under that snow for hours, although it could not have been more than seconds as my father plunged in and pulled me out.

I often remember this event when thinking about my diagnosis of Asperger's syndrome. Feeling my father's hand grasping the back of my T-shirt and hauling me out into the sunshine is very like the day my psychologist told me I was on the autism spectrum. From that moment, I began to make sense of the difficulties I had always experienced, to piece together a way to live my life. For me, the neurotypical world is still as unnavigable as that Colorado snowdrift, but I am beginning to draft a map that will help me chart my course.

Routines have always been important to me. Whenever possible, I do the same things in the same order for the same length of time. I wear the same clothes (making multiple purchases of items I like to wear), eat the same foods, do the same hobbies. I try not to worry that this behaviour is unusual by neurotypical standards; repetition is calming and helps me to keep equilibrium, as other areas of my life, such as work, are not so easy to order. There are times when I can't follow my daily routine, but I have put into place strategies to manage the stress this inevitably causes.

More than disruptions to routine, interactions with people are an enormous source of stress for me. I rarely know what to say in any given situation and find that I take what is said at face value, unable to infer meanings, which often frustrates neurotypical speakers. I find it very challenging to be in conversation with more than one participant. The talk ping-pongs around; I am never sure who will speak next and when it will be my turn to say something. Even now, I do not know how to join groups of people at a meeting or party, and when I do find myself in a group, I don't pick up on the signal that they are going to disperse – discovering myself standing alone with everyone gone!

As a result of these trials, I limit my exposure to neurotypical events, one per week as a maximum where possible and keep my time spent in a social situation short – 2 hours is my absolute limit. I have a small group of people with whom I feel comfortable, people who understand my need for clear communication and are happy to spend time in silence as well. It helps that these people like to engage in the activities I enjoy and are happy for me to retreat if feeling overwhelmed. I also find friendship and support in online forums for people on the autism spectrum.

Food shopping is a sensory nightmare – over-lit, overstocked supermarkets clogged with people, trollies and children conspire to overwhelm me so I have learned to go during quiet periods. I always take a list, organised according to the store layout. The self-scan and pack system is useful as I don't have to engage with a cashier. Buying clothes is another ordeal and one which I conquer by shopping online. I can search for the items I need, filtering them according to colour, fabric and size. I can try the items on in the comfort of my own home and return those that are not suitable.

I am fortunate that I have found a job that suits my need for routine and is limited in the need to deal with people. Managing a database plays to my skills; it requires attention to detail, accuracy and focus. I am more than happy to undertake repetitive tasks and often perform data analysis, which I really enjoy. I work in a very small office that is quiet, calm and has muted lighting. Perfume is my biggest issue at work. I can tolerate light, fresh scents but musky perfumes are simply too strong. I counter this by using a coconut hand cream and rubbing a small amount under my nostrils. It is not perfect, but I do find that the smell of perfume lessens as the day goes on.

With all the challenges of living in a neurotypical world, it is important for me to have an array of strategies for stress and anxiety reduction. Every day I must take time to decompress. I need to retreat into the sanctuary that is my peaceful, uncluttered home with its neutral colour scheme and lack of strong smells or bright lights. I like to enjoy the sound of silence or quiet talk radio. I read during this time or crochet, a wonderfully repetitive and rhythmic activity.

I often think I should take shares in a camomile tea producer as I drink such a lot of it! The camomile has a calming effect but, more than that, the ritual of making tea, as the Chinese have known for centuries, is relaxing in itself. Even holding a warm cup – I have a smooth-surfaced pottery mug with a handle that is just the right size – is restorative.

I practise Qigong, a form of Tai Chi, for 20 minutes every morning. Slow movements, coupled with the focus on deep, 'belly' breathing, relax the body during practice but the effects of the Qigong continue throughout the day as I find myself pausing to breathe or focus on a physical task. This mindfulness calms my thoughts and brings me into the present moment; I am so often living in the past or worrying about the future. Ten minutes of meditation follows my Qigong practise. I try to clear my mind and remember that thoughts are simply that – just thoughts.

Walking is another activity that alleviates stress for me. I am sure my neighbours think I am mad as I follow the same 30-minute route each day, rain or shine.

I find that I am sensitive to sugar and additives in food. My stress and anxiety are much worse if the things I eat are processed, so I enjoy a 'clean' diet. I eat little and often to maintain an optimum blood sugar level.

I ensure that I always carry a kit with a set of headphones, hand-sanitiser (the thought of germs causes me a great deal of stress), coconut hand cream to mask strong smells, snacks and water. With my kit, I can manage most sensory issues and if I can't, I give myself permission to leave.

With careful organisation and planning, I am mostly able to keep my stress and anxiety under control. I operate under the motto KISS: Keep it simple, stupid! While I'd love to be a captain of an industry or a high-flying politician, I now accept that I have limits. After all, a successful life is a life well lived, and by taking care of the Asperger's needs I have, I am finding that I am getting more pleasure from doing less, with less stress.

## David's story: 'Everything is different but nothing has changed'

I always felt different and remember thinking I'd been dropped by a spaceship and one day they would come and collect me. For a number of years as a child, I got really interested in astronomy and put my bed by the window so I could look up at the stars. I didn't fit in school; I was always the last to be picked in team games, and at play time you'd find me standing on my own by the fence, or I just sat and read a book in the library. I was bullied by both pupils and staff but I was good at maths and sciences. In an English lesson, one homework assignment was to write an essay on 'The humour of Jane Austen'. My essay was very short but very honest and I wrote, 'There is no humour, she's not funny'. The teacher's response was to get angry, give me a detention, send me to the headmaster and afterwards mimic me – I thought she was unfair as I was only giving my honest answer.

I've seen counsellors and therapists over the years who mainly diagnosed me as having a social phobia and depression. They explained that social phobia was being scared of what people were thinking of you and worried that you would make a mistake. That wasn't my experience, but I couldn't explain what it was that made me unable to communicate with strangers. I also had some sensory issues such as being overwhelmed by loud noise, bright lights and uncomfortable clothes.

Despite everything, I eventually got married to a very caring lady called Claire who worked as a nurse. I had a job in IT as a customer service engineer for a large company. I was surprisingly successful and won regional and national prizes, although I always avoided Christmas parties, trips to the pub or firm's days out. To me the work was problem solving – all very logical and binary. People would ring in with an IT problem and it was simply a question of analysis and diagnosis. I would ask questions and they would answer yes or no – no middle ground, no shades of grey, no complicated emotions. I was so successful that I was promoted to team lead and given managerial responsibilities – that's where it all started to go wrong. I couldn't cope with understanding other people's issues and conflicts and I got depressed and ended up in a psychiatric hospital – which was a nightmare. Claire had read an article on autism and discussed it with the psychiatrist who made a referral.

Eventually, after a long wait, I saw a psychologist who carried out a detailed autism/Asperger's assessment. He went through my whole life history, seemed to understand and had a questionnaire completed by my mother. Claire was present and I remember her holding my hand a couple of times. It was a relief when he said that I'd got autism, but no great surprise. However, I was surprised at how emotional I was; Claire hugged me and I felt a tear on my cheek as I shook hands with the psychologist – I felt that I'd got an answer at last.

From that moment onwards, everything was different although nothing obviously changed. I felt as if somebody had turned the lights on. I thought and dreamed vividly about my past and all the incidents that could now be explained by my condition. It was like I was re-experiencing my life through the prism of autism. I told a few people and generally got a good reaction although I felt my sister and her husband scrutinising me – leaving me feeling a little self-conscious. The best reaction was from my manager at work who surprisingly said, 'I feel honoured that you've told me'. With the help of HR, we managed to restructure my job so I was without any managerial responsibilities – earning less money, but I didn't care – it felt like a great improvement.

I think getting the diagnosis 6 years ago has stabilised my life. I saw the psychologist who helped me unravel what was the autism and what was depression. It helped me unravel who and why I am. I still see that psychologist about once every 9 months which helps as I know there is someone out there who would understand me if the stresses build up. As I read in a book once, I see the diagnosis as a signpost not a label. It indicated where

I've come from and gives me some direction of where I'm going. Claire has helped enormously – she is my social eyes and ears – I would struggle without her. I must be difficult to live with as I don't really like going out much and don't like holidays. Claire said, 'Why don't we go to the Grand Canyon for your birthday?' My reaction was, 'It's just a big ditch, what's the point, why don't we watch the video?' I'd rather stay at home for a week, go running, play my guitar, work on the house and garden and on my birthday watch a film and have a takeaway pizza. The diagnosis has helped me accept who I am and helped me to stop 'trying to be normal' and doing things that I don't want to do. Everything has changed but nothing is different.

## Rachel's story: 'Diagnosis has been a gift'

I was always a quiet and solitary child, although I didn't want to be, and at times, the loneliness was overwhelming. I had a very abusive home life so I escaped into books and solitude and created my own imaginary world. I used to stim (repetitive hand flapping) regularly and was noted as being odd, but it was blamed on my mother's mental illness. Friends were few and far between, but after about age 8, I was able to maintain a solid friendship with another child whose father had terminal cancer. She was used to the unusual and was able to be friends with me. When I was 18, I made another friend who taught me the basics of social skills, such as the value of asking questions and listening for answers.

My daughter was diagnosed as autistic at age 4, but it had been apparent since she was 2. But because she was so similar to me, I did not understand the concerns. Once she was diagnosed, I realised that autism is written about differently to the way I experience it. I 'do what I do'. I am me. So, to see my behaviour and personality presented as wrong, abnormal and dysfunctional was very isolating. For example, as an adult, I am quite gregarious and like being with people up to a point, but socialising is exhausting and I can only manage a certain amount, and then I need my space. I do occasionally make the odd social slip up, but by and large, I can usually unpick social situations. I count seconds of eye contact, closely mimic others and have to plan conversations. It always surprises me that other people are so bothered about clothes and make-up. I don't think I'm stuck in rigid routines; this does not fit my experience.

Before the assessment, I had to fill in questionnaires and give one to my mother which proved to be quite difficult. She kept on saying, 'Oh it doesn't look good, does it Rachel?' Her experience was so different to mine as I saw getting a diagnosis as a positive thing. I'd hoped it might relieve some of her guilt as I was such an odd child (flapping hands, singing myself to sleep whilst rocking my head, didn't walk until I was two and had no friends). I'd hoped for understanding and possibly some healing with Mum, but that was not to be.

The assessment was really thorough and took about 3 hours. I remember a very sweaty seat and counting the bricks repetitively on a building opposite the clinician's office. They made a particularly interesting pattern around some windows in groups of seven – my favourite number to count to. I was really surprised to get a full diagnosis of autistic spectrum disorder (Asperger's syndrome) as I expected to be diagnosed with just having traits. When it was over, I phoned my other half and said, 'Guess what, I'm autistic!' He answered; 'So what's new?' and that was that, no drama, just carrying on. I was quite disorientated after 3 hours and had to work out what way to walk. I felt quite vulnerable and frightened as I suddenly twigged that I simply can't hide that I struggle so much socially any more. I bumped into a man I knew who had two autistic twins and told him about my diagnosis, and he said something jocular like, 'So you're a nutter now too'. I enjoyed the light-heartedness of it as it stopped me from brooding. I managed to navigate myself home on the bus and hugged my children. I also wrote a message on Facebook informing all my friends that I'd got the diagnosis, and that I wasn't about to start hiding, and although I knew I was as mad as a box of frogs, I was still part of this world and intended to stay so. Gratifyingly, everyone who posted was hugely supportive and several just posted 'Croak', which made me smile lots. I felt so honoured that people were prepared to stay with me. I've also realised that socialising on Facebook suits me much better than face-to-face contact as it's much less exhausting and it gives you much more time to work out the social rules.

Now, 2 years later, I think that an autism diagnosis is the gift that keeps on giving! I am not sure how I would have felt if I had been given it as a child, as the emphasis seems to be on the negatives. It would have been lovely for someone to say to me: 'It's OK not to be social, you can trust yourself and follow your special interest'. But, when I was younger, I felt I needed to be a more well-rounded person, based on the many personal criticisms and bullying I received. I have learned mindfulness and feel more in charge of the way I respond to my thoughts. I also still take a low-dose selective serotonin reuptake inhibitor (SSRI) which helps with the anxiety arising from my sensory processing disorder. This helps me be a better parent as I really struggle with the noise that the children make.

Knowing I am autistic has freed me to be myself. I can rejoice in being quirky and different as I actually am. It is great knowing that it is the shape of my brain that determines this, as opposed to me being a dunce and wilfully not understanding stuff. It's great to embrace the huge feeling of joy and love my special interest engulfs me in, and enjoy it just for that, instead of berating myself for not pushing it further. It is great to understand more about sensory issues and use them to my advantage – long walks in the woods, weighted blankets and just the right music for my mood. It's wonderful to finally understand what sort of person I am.

The gifts it's given me as a parent are immense. I will share my children's special interests; I WON'T stop them stimming. I love them for being their quirky selves and best of all I can choose to present their unique neurology as a positive. I never understood why society makes such a fuss about difference – I suffer from face blindness and struggle to recognise people. Most people seem to run with the crowd for their protection which makes them practically invisible to me. Difference means I can see them and this should be celebrated. Difference is not a threat to the crowd but an added dimension to humanity.

## Floyd's story: 'My role models are James Bond and Bertie Wooster'

Throughout my life, people have said, 'Why can't you just be normal?'. I have always accepted that there is a misalignment between myself and the rest of the world. This, however, has never given me the feeling of being a lesser person; in fact, it has always been the opposite. I have grown up with the permanent frustration that the majority of people simply do not work correctly, but that is the way of the world. While attempting to blend in, I have developed an overconfidence in who I am. This belief has allowed me to survive disappointment, job sacking, relationship breakdown and social faux pas.

I have spent my life watching people, learning social norms and rules, imitating social manners and etiquette. I have learnt to be a successful salesman. There are rules to selling which centre around placing the other person in a position where they have no alternative but to buy. I have learned to suppress certain emotional reactions that, when displayed, have appeared to others childlike in their over-animation.

I have taken on a persona that is a combination of the fictitious characters James Bond and Bertie Wooster because both characters are funny, stylish and popular. Both characters have been special interests of mine since I was very young, and I have all their books and films. I have created a socially acceptable self and now survive as a fashionista – I love wearing unusual colourful fashionable clothing. I have developed a cool steely persona that cannot be hurt but is also very charming and funny and that, by using self-deprecating humour where I am the object of ridicule, I gain popularity.

The diagnosis explained why there had always been a misalignment and, in a way, set me free to be myself rather than emulating the reactions of others. I enjoy being the Bertie Wooster/James Bond character and would feel lost not having them as the blueprint to my life, as this has also given me a love of England, culture, antiques and fine clothing.

For the past 20 years, I have used my neurotypical wife as a template or guide for the social norm, rather than my juvenile excitable outbursts of emotion. I have noted that she never discusses her personal emotions or reveals them in an exuberant manner and feels that discussing them in public makes her vulnerable, and so I have adopted this. However, it has resulted in a burying of my emotions so deep it has taken me some intense effort to retrieve them again. In an attempt to understand the benefits of her working this way, I have quizzed her relentlessly over the years. She has claimed that my relentless quizzing has made her depressed as she does not know why she works this way. I operate so differently than her in the sense that I am much more rational and less emotional. For example, she would get jealous if I was friendly with another woman, or she would want repeated reassurance that I love her. I just don't see the need – I have told her I love her on many occasions – why the need for such repetition?

To be honest, our marriage has struggled and failed particularly since my diagnosis, where she has become depressed and unhappy, saying, 'The person I married isn't the person I thought he was'. She says she wants me to 'get better and be normal', saying, 'You're too logical, not emotional enough', rather than accepting me for who I was. We are now separated at her request as she has found romance with somebody at her work whom she says is 'more empathic'. I have finally achieved the cathartic experience of crying, which I have enjoyed very much. Wallowing in sadness has been strangely satisfying; however, I am not able to dwell on these emotions for long as my strong logical brain kicks in and tells me that I have had enough and puts them away again.

Since our separation, I have had to develop a social life away from my wife, and the freedom of the diagnosis has allowed me to revert back to the colourful character that I was 20 years ago. I have discovered that the majority of people find my gregarious, overzealous nature refreshing and people are accepting of me when I explain that my exuberance is a result of the fact that my brain is wired up differently and that autism is not a thing to be feared.

I purposely seek out other autistic people and want to inspire them to believe in themselves, suggesting they have been gifted with an insight to do great things and explaining the advantages of being able to control how they feel with the power of their logical minds. Emotions have a purpose but, in my view, neurotypical people have emotions in abundance and are controlled by them. The diagnosis has set me free to be myself and not feel bad about it!

## Melanie's story: 'It validated me – I'm more autistic militant now'

The experience of getting a diagnosis has made me more autistic militant. Instead of hiding it and thinking that I'm just odd, I'm more likely to stand up for myself and my rights. I will enjoy my sensory sensitivities – things I really enjoy – like swimming in the river, standing with my toes in squishy mud, listening to the rustling of a tree, feeling the leather on the steering wheel of my car, seeing rainbows and waterfalls. I will ask for a quiet table in a restaurant; I will tell somebody pushing against me and squashing into me on the tube to keep away; and I will flap my hands at work when I am stressed.

I had a disciplinary at work before the diagnosis, and they said I was 'bullying a colleague', but in my view, I was just being honest, telling her straight, albeit I am a bit too blunt. Now I have told my fellow nurses at work: 'I've got autism so I won't know if you're unhappy or cross unless you start crying or shouting, so you will have to tell me. If you see me being inappropriate or getting stressed, just tell me'. The young nurses are great and just accept me and the situation, but the older ones can be a bit difficult. I know we all have to fit in and it is a compromise between the autistic and neurotypical worlds, but I don't suppress or rein it in as much. Before I used to think I was odd – as a child I used to think that I was a fairy child although my parents did not think so – now I feel validated and I'm happier being me.

My sister said, 'That explains why you had temper tantrums when anyone sat in your chair at the table or you wouldn't wear wool or you'd go out in a summer dress in the snow in winter'.

## Gerry's story: 'I still feel angry … I'll never catch up'

Wednesday, 1 October 2017, another date to add to my ever-growing collection of memorable/unforgettable dates. This date may offer an explanation as to why dates play such an important part in my life and why I remember every significant date. This is the date I was diagnosed with Asperger's syndrome/autism.

The Asperger's diagnosis came as a surprise to me and my family. I initially refused an assessment, but it was eventually taken out of my hands when I was sectioned under the Mental Health Act. To be taken off the section, I had to agree to be referred for an assessment.

I feel angry about having the diagnosis of Asperger's. I am angry that I now have a diagnosis that I don't know what to do with. I am angry that I'm angry. I don't like being angry; anger is something that terrifies me. I'm angry when people say, 'Albert Einstein had Asperger's', because I'm not Albert Einstein. I don't have any special talents; I'm not a genius; and I'm fed up with hearing about it.

My initial thoughts following the diagnosis were 'it must be wrong. I can't have Asperger's'. This is still one of the most dominant feelings that I have. I am struggling to settle the diagnosis in my own mind. The more I read about Asperger's, the more things make sense: my love of routine and order, my strong belief about right and wrong, my strong dislike of change, my social difficulties and sensitivity to touch. All of it fits, yet I can't seem to accept the diagnosis.

The diagnosis, though unwanted, has in a way provided a form of relief. It helps provide an explanation to some of my quirks and also helps my friends and family understand parts of my, sometimes strange, behaviour.

I have always had strong thoughts about what I should achieve to become a successful and worthy person. I set myself targets to reach by certain birthdays – by age 25, I wanted to be in full-time employment, own my own car and be living independently. By age 30, I wanted to be in a relationship, progressing in my job and looking to buy my own home. Now at 29 all but one of the targets have been missed. I own my own car – my dream car. The Asperger's diagnosis has made me question whether I will ever be able to reach these targets. It has made me question whether I will ever be the person that I want to be. The diagnosis has made me realise that I need to re-evaluate my aims and reconstruct my hopes for the future. Before the diagnosis, I had accepted/realised that I was different from my friends/peers, but a part of me had always thought I would catch up, at some point something would click. The diagnosis makes me feel like this is unlikely to ever happen – it has taken away some hope. It is unlikely that I will ever catch up or be the person I want to be.

Although the diagnosis may potentially answer some questions, it also raises a lot of new ones. Overall, I still have very mixed feelings about the Asperger's diagnosis. Now I have had time to digest the diagnosis, I am able to see some positives and understand why it was important to have the assessment.

## Max's Story: 'I was a hermit … now I try and live in the real world'

My life was always quite challenging, but I thought I was OK in primary school, as I kept to my small group of friends from a small, close-knit housing estate where everyone knew each other and connections were easily built and maintained. All that changed when I started secondary school, which was a bus journey away, not a short walk down the road. I was torn away from my comfort zone and felt traumatised. Due to my quietness, I was put through a special needs class. I scored 100% in their test, so they naively decided I didn't need any help. I was being picked on for almost everything, including being quiet, and mostly ended up sitting on my own. Eventually, my attendance dropped and I was only attending classes that interested me.

I attended college for a year, studying music technology, and got a distinction for my academic work. I specialised in Elvis Presley between 1953 and 1956 – the period when he left school, signed for Sun Records and then signed for RCA in New York. I know all the records he made and who played on them. I tried to play guitar but was rubbish as I couldn't play with the other members of the group – I was out of sync, couldn't interact with them and was told my guitar playing was 'robotic'.

I dropped out of college and became a hermit for a couple of years. I would never leave the house, staying in my bedroom, usually with the curtains drawn. I grew my hair and nails and really didn't look after myself. My interests were also quite narrow; I loved my music and video games and would become obsessed with the story and the characters. I even built websites dedicated to my favourites. I made friends on the internet because I could join message boards dedicated to subjects that I was interested in. Writing is so much easier than speaking.

Eventually, I pushed myself out of the house, to meet a girl that I'd met online. Playing video games was good, but I craved human interaction outside. I fell in love with Mandy and soon moved in with her and her parents. She had everything in common with me, so it was much easier to connect with her. Even better, we had broken the ice on the internet, so I didn't have to suffer with any of the small talk. However, I was extremely uncomfortable with her family and would hide away in her room during the day, when she went to work.

I had always suspected I had autism and eventually reached the breaking point where I had to get help to find out if my suspicions were correct.

I eventually got an appointment to see a psychologist. I was absolutely terrified, but after a few hours, I was diagnosed. I was so happy; I finally understood why I had acted this way all of my life.

It was liberating. A few months later, I was invited along to a few support sessions, where I was able to meet other adults who had also been diagnosed. We all sat in a waiting room, and it was actually great to see people tapping their feet, biting their nails and flapping their hands and fingers. It was great to see people who acted the same way I did and felt the same way I did in these situations – I was not alone.

The diagnosis did change my life. I am more comfortable in myself because I know the reason why I act in certain ways. Mandy accepted my diagnosis and has been very supportive – I think she is a little bit 'on the spectrum' herself. We have our own flat now and I have a job as a cleaner, which I really enjoy. I'm good at it because I like the routine, regularity and structure and I'm on my own. I only wish that my condition had been spotted earlier on in life, as I might have got help in school and wouldn't have spent all those years in my bedroom as a hermit.

Being in the real world is my main difficulty. I am fine on my own or with Mandy, but if I go on a train or in a coffee shop, I have my iPod on or wear my sunglasses. I know I have got to get a balance between being in the real world and being in my own world. If I go into a coffee shop, I try not to wear my iPod all the time and try to make some small talk with the person serving rather than just saying 'Cappuccino please'.

## Julia's story: 'If I had known earlier, I might have saved my job'

It is frightening when you feel different and I've always felt different, almost as if I spoke a different language to everybody else. As a child, I'd say things wrong and I'd have no idea what I'd done – I had a complete blind spot. I am unaware of how I appear to others because it's difficult to see things from their point of view. I just saw people recoiling from me. Friendships were a struggle to initiate and maintain. I always knew the issue lay with me as I just didn't know what to say. It's like everybody else seemed to 'know'; they had a handbook or script and I hadn't been given one. I have got better over the years and one key turning point was practising smiling and saying hello when greeting people.

The diagnosis was an epiphany, a turning point in my life and answered about 50 years' worth of questions. Afterwards, I spent a lot of time reinterpreting things that had happened to me, with a lot of 'if only' regrets. Suddenly there was an explanation for the gaffes and misunderstandings over the years. I have wounds and deep scars inflicted by people as they have reacted to my autism. All the unpleasantness can now be put down to something other than my flawed moral character. I am not a bad person after all – it wasn't my fault. Many people whom I have known over the years – colleagues, parents and siblings have formed an opinion about me which has not always been complimentary. It is difficult to explain to them that I do have a problem, but it's not what they thought it was.

I started to meet with other Aspies and really did feel at home for the first time – I felt included and accepted by that group. We would share our common experiences, and there was a lot of head nodding and reassurance. We are all very different and don't conform to any stereotype, but underneath, there is something that we all have in common.

Perhaps my greatest regret is that I didn't follow up my initial encounter with the concept of Asperger's syndrome, which I read about in an article in 'New Scientist' in April 2001. The article, by Professor Simon Baron-Cohen, proposed a list of ten questions, and invited anyone who could answer 'yes' to all ten to write in and take part in his research. I had eight 'yes' and two possibles. I didn't take it any further at the time because I worried that if I took the article to my GP, he would just tell me to stop wasting time.

Two years ago, I was made redundant from my job as an engineer – I was a woman in a man's world. I feel that if I'd have had the diagnosis earlier, I might have done better at work and saved my career. Unfortunately, I got a diagnosis a year after losing my job. They were making redundancies and I was told 'You don't fit in', which was probably right, but very upsetting to hear. I know that I was one of the better engineers and always got on with the job and produced good work, but I didn't have any allies or friends at work. I couldn't do superficial small talk and my direct, rather blunt, but always honest, manner put me on the wrong side of office politics.

I used to get angry if people interrupted me after I'd said a few words, thinking they knew what I meant, but in fact they didn't and they'd take the conversation off in a direction I didn't intend and I'd have to drag it back again. Or they would 'interpret' what I said, drawing inferences, which again I didn't intend. I have a deep need to work out how the world works, so I ended up asking questions – too many questions. I want to understand things. I am very intolerant of ambiguity, and if things are not clear, it feels as if everything is going to fall apart. Having the diagnosis means that

I have legal rights and have a legal disability which means I would have been entitled to 'reasonable adjustments' in the workplace and maybe I'd still be there today.

I am very glad that I got the diagnosis, as it has been a great help – knowing that my difficulties have a biological basis makes them much easier to deal with. I carry a card around in my wallet in case I get into difficult situations. The message says something like, 'Please don't take it personally if my behaviour seems odd; I'm autistic and don't express myself very well in unfamiliar situations'.

Although initially I was relieved, my feelings gradually changed and I became angrier that I wasn't diagnosed earlier and there was a sense of frustration at being misunderstood for much of my life. But I'd much rather be angry than confused and depressed!

# CHAPTER 5

# Processing information

## *Cognition, language and sensory issues*

## Uneven cognitive, language and sensory profiles

This chapter could be construed as three chapters in one, as it will combine an exploration of autistic cognition (thinking), language and sensory issues. The reason for the amalgamation is because all the three areas are about how our brains process information. More importantly, it's about how an autistically designed brain often produces an exceptionally uneven, spiky profile of skills – characterised by extreme peaks and troughs, strengths and vulnerabilities. For example, on cognitive tasks involving visual search or identifying perceptual patterns, such as *Embedded Figures and Block Design*, autistic people are often above average – although not always. However, on tasks involving speed of processing information, verbal comprehension or executive functioning, such as *Wisconsin Card Sorting Test*, scores tend to be lower than average (Xie et al, 2020). This explains why school pupils with this uneven profile of academic abilities may be misdiagnosed as having a learning disability. This diversity means that it is sensible to exercise extreme caution when making generalisations or talking about concepts such as overall intelligence. For example, Temple Grandin, as a child, was initially going to be sent to an institution for people with a learning disability but ended up becoming an academic professor. Similarly, Albert Einstein was considered rather 'backwards' because he didn't speak until he was 6 years old but he went on to win a Nobel prize. This contrast in extreme abilities may be seen in the areas of language; an autistic person with an above average vocabulary might struggle to understand the meaning of a simple idiom or proverb. Furthermore, in sensory areas an autistic person with a highly developed musical sense, perhaps having perfect pitch, might struggle to filter out distracting background noises.

## Attention – single channel?

There are three types of attention: (1) sustained attention, which means concentrating on one thing for a long period of time; (2) divided or split attention, which means concentrating on two things at the same time and (3) switching attention, meaning, switching attention backwards and forwards between different items or stimuli. Autistic individuals are often remarkably good at sustained attention, which can be a real strength, but not so good at divided attention or switching attention. However, this sustained attention and ability to process information depends on how the information is presented. Autistic people are often superior at processing information if it is static or concrete, with factual details being presented sequentially through one channel. Conversely, they may struggle with processing more complex or dynamic bits of information presented simultaneously in pieces, through multiple channels.

The autistic brain is often remarkably good at attending to detail, having an 'eagle eye' for spotting details that it is interested in. It's as if the person is looking at the world through a rolled-up piece of paper, a single channel, but often not seeing the wider picture. Sometimes people are able to concentrate or sustain attention for a considerable amount of time, almost in a trance-like state, oblivious to external stimulation. One example was Nick, a computer coder/programmer who said, 'I can hyperfocus and sometimes spend 10 hours a day working on a piece of code without taking a break for food or drink. I don't notice my body or anything around me. Afterwards I'm exhausted and need to sleep'. However, if the autistic person is not interested in the subject, they often have a problem filtering out extraneous background stimulation or information and are therefore easily distracted. For many, it's an 'off–on' switch – fully invested or not interested at all. A common difficulty in people with autism is maintaining joint/divided attention and switching between tasks or attending to multiple cues. Frequently people will say,

- I find it difficult to look at you and talk at the same time.

- I find it difficult to listen and take notes at the same time in a lecture.

- I'm not very good at thinking and talking at the same time.

- I don't like subtitled films because I have to read, look and listen all at once.

This one channel autistic thinking is illustrated by Alex's comment:

> I'm a real single channel person, so bad at multitasking that when I'm watching TV, I completely zone out of everything else. If the phone rings I don't hear it. If my flatmate comes into my room to give me a message, they have to stand in front of the TV before I realise, they're saying something to me! People get so cross but I can't help it. I really don't like being interrupted, because then I feel I have to start again.

# Executive functioning – flexibility and seeing the big picture

Executive skills are all the tasks that a chief executive officer (CEO) of a large organisation needs, or the conductor of an orchestra or a general marshalling his troops. At the heart of these skills is a mental flexibility, an ability to see the big picture, to organise and plan, hold information in the mind and switch and divide attention, being flexible enough to change plans. These skills are thought to be located in the frontal lobes of the brain, and human beings have large well-developed frontal lobes, unlike animals further down the evolutionary scale. It could be argued that human civilisation has expanded at the same rate as mankind's frontal lobes have evolved.

The skills of a good CEO, or any executive, include the following:

- Seeing the overall 'bigger picture' – taking a broad or different perspective.

- Multitasking by flexibly switching and dividing attention.

- Planning and organising – thinking ahead, imagining the future.

- Setting goals and organising ways to achieve those goals.

- Recognising mistakes and flexibly changing plans if necessary.

- Prioritising what is most important.

- Summarising and not getting caught up in details.

- Making decisions.

- Problem solving and abstract reasoning.

- Managing time and deadlines successfully.

It might be that the autistic person is less effective at being a CEO, conductor or general but excels as a specialist: the virtuoso violinist, a backroom technician or the skilled rifleman.

Felicity, a client of mine, stands out as one of the best examples of somebody with poor executive skills, but a great eye for detail. She was 18 years old when initially referred by a psychiatrist who had diagnosed her with depression. It transpired that Felicity wasn't really depressed but was highly anxious and had undiagnosed autism. She was highly intelligent and achieved four A*s in her A levels and been accepted to study at Cambridge University. Her mother and I anticipated numerous social problems, sensory issues and difficulties with changed routine so we wrote various letters to the University's Special Needs Department, her tutor and mentor, who all made various *'reasonable adjustments'*. She was provided with a special quiet en suite room, which she did not have to vacate in holiday times like the other students, and was even allowed to take her pet iguana.

However, problems arose that we didn't anticipate. One was that Felicity struggled with writing academic essays because this involved planning, identifying key points, giving opinions and writing a coherent argument. She could remember and regurgitate individual facts, which is why she had done so well at A level but was less able to make abstract connections, i.e. identifying the main ideas and minor details, making summaries, metaphysically hovering over the project and seeing the overall picture – like a helicopter hovering over a landscape when the pilot is able to see the lie-of-the-land. Felicity invariably got sucked into the details and became lost in an academic maze. The ability to write a university essay requires a different style of thinking – executive thinking – than the thinking required in school. If she had been given a multiple-choice exam, just testing her knowledge, she would have passed with flying colours.

It turned out that Felicity's devoted mother ended up being her 'executive secretary', helping her plan, organise, structure, connect, summarise and prioritise information while flexibly making changes and moving things around in her university essays. In essence, her mother was taking on the function of Felicity's frontal lobes. People on the autism spectrum often perform better if given external support, someone to give a reminder, a prompt, to 'boot up' those executive skills that are often dormant.

The following examples, given by clients, highlight other issues attributed to poor executive ability, particularly in the areas of time keeping, dealing with complex information and summarising key information.

- I hate writing essays as I struggle to structure and plan my thoughts on paper. I struggle over every sentence and don't know how to start or link things up. Sometimes I just launch in. It would be much better if I could just write down a list of bullet points about what I know.

- I'm a cleaner and have about eight areas to work in, but I struggle to judge and allocate time to each task. I ended up working many more hours than I was paid for. I'd get 'lost in a sea of time'. The strategy that was most helpful was setting my phone alarm to go off and alert me when it was time to switch tasks.

- I was top of my class on my software development course and was marked excellent on my first placement where there was a very specific job to do. In my second placement, I was promoted to Consultant Advisor for a large company but unfortunately failed. They presented me with numerous multifaceted problems and lots of raw data presented all at once rather than one piece at a time. If they had given me a single task to do, I could do it, but they gave me open-ended vague instructions, suggesting I 'use my initiative'. I realise I need clear specific guidelines, structured tasks and information presented singularly.

- As a senior nurse, I was involved in reporting on an investigation at work and had to produce a report. It took me ages to prepare and I kept going over the deadline. Eventually, I finished it and sent it to

*Table 5.1* Executive skills questions

| | |
|---|---|
| 1 | Do you have difficulty doing more than one thing at a time – multitasking? |
| 2 | Do you have difficulty deciding what is most important and what is least important – prioritising? |
| 3 | If there is an interruption, or unexpected change, can you very quickly switch back to what you were doing? |
| 4 | Do you have difficulty summarising information, or 'getting to the point'? |
| 5 | Do you concentrate more on the details rather than the whole picture? |
| 6 | Do you tend to take what people say very literally, sometimes missing out on subtle meanings? |
| 7 | Do you have difficulty organising your thoughts, either on paper or when speaking? |
| 8 | Do you need instructions spelt out specifically, in clear, simple, direct language? |
| 9 | Can you get so absorbed in a task that you lose track of time? |
| 10 | Do you have difficulties getting started, stopping or changing activities? |

my manager. He sent it back saying, 'This report should be 25 pages, you have sent me 140 pages! Too much detail, please cut down and summarise'. This is something I really struggle to do as it all seems equally important to me.

Identification of executive difficulties are scattered across the B2 and B3 criteria of the DSM-V. The questions above in Table 5.1 are designed to help identify key cognitive executive difficulties.

## Tips for improving executive skills

1 Stop, step back and don't rush into the details. Survey the situation.

2 Ask yourself questions: what, when, how, where, why and who? Decide on the main issues and identify the details. What would other people want me to achieve/include? What is my goal? If unsure, ask for help or clarification.

3 Make a plan to achieve your goal, identify steps or action points – write a list.

4 Self-monitor. Occasionally stand back, check and ask yourself questions: am I on course? What can I change? What are the other options?

5 Ask for advice and feedback from others – check out another person's perspective, ask for help.

## Memory – an 'eye for detail' and understanding 'savant' skills

For many years, clinicians and scientists have noted contradictory features of memory in those with an autism diagnosis. In 1943, Leo Kanner observed that, "the children's memory was phenomenal" (p245). They had an excellent memory for general knowledge, phenomenal ability to rote learn poems, names and the precise recollection of complex patterns and sequences. On the television quiz programme *The Chase (2009–present)*, the chaser, known as *The Governess*, Anne Hegerty, who is autistic, demonstrates a phenomenal general knowledge memory. By contrast, a meta-analysis of academic memory studies in autism, carried out by Desaunnay (2020), showed that autistic people had greater difficulty with short-term memory (working memory) compared to a non-autistic group, and there was a small difference in long-term verbal memory and a medium difference in visual memory, when compared to non-autistic groups.

A good example of extreme skills and weaknesses in memory was illustrated by Felicity, the young Cambridge University student, discussed in the previous section. In her first year, she had great difficulty finding her way from her room to the lecture theatre block, which was a short walk along the ancient paved stoned streets of Cambridge. Her sense of direction was extremely poor and she would often get lost. When asked how she tried to remember the route, she commented, 'I will look at the cracks in the paving stones, or count the paving stones, and look out for the daffodils'. I asked, 'What if the daffodils were out of season?' to which she replied, 'I'd still be able to see the stalks'. Felicity was great on the small miniscule detail but not very good at standing back and perceiving the overall picture or holding in mind a mental map or spatial memory of the streets of Cambridge. Felicity also had a problem with remembering faces (prosopagnosia) and often remembered people by a detail such as their hair. Her mother related a story about picking Felicity up from school one day after having had a haircut and Felicity not recognising her in the school playground, being unable to pick her out from the other mothers because of her change in appearance.

Occasionally an autistic person might even have a photographic memory with the ability to recall accurately scenes or whole pages of a book. Pupils with autism are sometimes wrongly accused of cheating in exams because they can reproduce, almost exactly, long pages of text from textbooks. One young man, Jermaine, was criticised by his teacher for not writing careful notes to study for his examination. He commented,

> I didn't write notes like everybody else, partly because my handwriting was so poor, but also because I didn't need to, as I could remember everything without writing it down. I could visualise all the information from the textbook. My teacher would be constantly criticising me and moaning to my parents, but in the end, I got an A* in the exam.

For most of us, this is not a recommended study technique! However, paradoxically, even though autistic people might have an excellent rote memory for learning and storing information, they can very often be forgetful when it comes to remembering to do things in the future. This is a slightly different type of memory called 'prospective memory', which involves holding something in the mind to do in the future (e.g. I must ring my mother this evening), while at the same time getting on with everyday life. Prospective memory involves doing two things simultaneously and is more an 'executive ability' than pure memory.

Less than 10% of autistic individuals have 'a degree of savant skill' or a photographic memory with an exceptional ability to recall details, but this process can provide insight into autistic memory. Synder (2012) suggests that this savant-like state is a pure form of autism, a mind that builds from parts to a whole, gets sucked into detail, has weak central coherence and limited ToM. There are people like the artist Steven Wiltshire, creator of photo-realistic cityscapes, who have photographic memories. He was once flown past the Houses of Parliament in a helicopter and produced a highly detailed accurate drawing of all the windows and turrets from memory. Synder's theory is that there is an atypical hemisphere imbalance or brain dysfunction in the left anterior temporal lobe, which is being compensated for by the right hemisphere's visual and spatial skills. Synder suggests that the left anterior temporal lobe is responsible for concept formation, packaging and labelling, assembling unprocessed raw information into wholes or holistic labels. If that area is damaged, either by a physical injury, a dementia (of the frontotemporal type) or left hemisphere stroke, these savant-like skills can be released and appear. It is as if the poorly functioning left hemisphere allows the right hemisphere, with its visual and perceptual skills, to be enhanced and take centre stage. Skills associated with savant-like abilities include having hyperlexia – a precocious reading ability as a young child. In hyperlexia, the child learns to read very quickly, remembers how to write and say the word, but doesn't actually understand the meaning of what they are reading. One man described that as a child he was able to read the newspapers fluently before starting school, but he didn't really understand what he was reading.

Marita, a young lady who was training to be a doctor, related an unusual, but telling, story:

> I have a photographic memory. I can remember every day of my life and can tell you what I was wearing, what I was eating, what I did and where I sat – it's really very annoying. If I read a sign walking around a National Trust property, I can't help but memorise it. I've read all the Harry Potter books at least 10 times and have read Matilda over 80 times. I was sitting on a train staring into space rereading the fifth Harry Potter book in my mind without the actual book and a lady opposite asked me what I was doing. I said, 'I'm reading Harry Potter'. To which she said, 'But where's the book dear?' My stupid memory is very useful in exams and was very good when I was a proof-reader but it is really annoying! Strangely my memory for routes is awful and I struggle to find the way to the local supermarket.

A further area of memory where autistic people often struggle is autobiographical memory, or memories about their own personal experiences. The person might remember 'facts' or semantic information, such as dates or times, or what they were wearing, but are less likely to remember the feelings associated with events. Consequently, there isn't that 'emotional carry over' from the past. This can contribute to a lower than average clarity of self-concept, or lack of sense of self and identity, which can be a feature of autistic people.

## Mathematics

About a quarter of autistic children are outstanding at mathematics and a quarter have real problems with it. Some have dyscalculia, which means they struggle to work out even the most basic mathematical concepts such as adding, subtracting or telling the time. While for others, mathematics is a strong subject because of the certainty associated with calculations and tables and the enjoyment in following rules and noticing details – if you know the correct answer you can prove it.

There are different types of maths as one client Ron illustrated,

> I was always good at pure maths at school and would get 98 per cent in exams and an A* at A level. But when I got to university, I had to do something called abstract maths and I just couldn't do it. I got 2 per cent in one exam. They would ask you to do things like prove that 1 is greater than 0. I couldn't think or imagine how to do it. I'm great with maths when there is a formula, a structured problem to solve, all straight lines and black and white. But abstract maths – no thanks! I dropped the maths degree at the end of the first year.

The following poem, posted on the Tony Attwood Asperger's website, captures well the understandable attraction between people with autism and numbers.

> *Numbers by David LeBlond*
>
> I like numbers
> they just add and subtract
> they don't hurt your feelings
> or overreact
> you can count on numbers
> to make things work out
> there's no second-guessing
> no worry or doubt
> numbers are my respite
> my port in the storm
> when the world is cruel and cold
> they are safe and warm

now they're not much to look at
(although eight is not bad)
they don't make you love them
or make you be sad
one thing about numbers
that won't be denied
they play by the rules
you cannot hide
if you make a mistake
or forget where you're at
they just won't forgive you
…we need people for that

## Language and communication: implied meaning: (pragmatics)

Autistic children frequently have late development of speech and a delay in both understanding and the development of verbal language. When we are babies, our world comprises sensory input and images, but we gradually acquire the use of language – there is a gradual transition from the sensory to verbal. This is the same for people with autism but the transition is often slower and more difficult and sometimes doesn't happen at all, resulting in what is known as 'autistic muteness'. But people without language can still communicate, although their language is based on sensory impressions, sounds, touch, taste, smells and images. Tito, a man diagnosed with autism, said, 'Words have no meaning; they are just noises like a dog barking'. Another client, Richard, explained, 'My first language is sensory, non-verbal. Every time I use a word, I'm using my second language. It's like I'm bilingual. I learned to speak by listening to the radio. That's why I sound like a (BBC) Radio 4 presenter'. In the past, autistic people with no or poor language skills were diagnosed as mentally retarded and sent to institutions, but we now know that often they have a form of autistic intelligence that is simply not based on words and language. This explains why sometimes people with autism will make up or invent idiosyncratic words (neologisms). These are often words that have a sensory onomatopoeic association with the object, such as 'clink' for a magnet and 'pinklipstar' for lipstick. Language skills improve over time and for most autistic people, difficulties would not be immediately obvious to an outsider, but they can still be there, under the surface, subtle and difficult to identify for the untrained eye.

Communicating is not just about language or words, but the ability to understand implied meaning – getting the gist or drift of a conversation. This is achieved by two means: (1) interpreting non-verbal messages and (2) by understanding that language can have dual meaning. Many autistic people are very precise in their choice of words, having wide vocabularies and perfectly enunciated words, but they still have trouble in some areas of communication. They have a lack of understanding of non-verbal signals implied by a look, a nod, a smile, a gesture, a tone of voice, a grunt etc. One client, Natasha, training to be a doctor in a busy hospital, illustrated this point well:

> If I'm going to understand people they need to speak directly, clearly and specifically to me, rather than making inferences. I was in the nurses' station the other day, with five other people, and the matron said, 'Someone's got to do that X-ray today', and raised her eyebrows, looking at me'. I really didn't know she was referring to me, so I didn't do the X-ray and got into trouble. Why didn't she just call me by name and tell me exactly and precisely what I had to do rather than having this mysterious code?

Language can be confusing if taken literally, because there are often hidden meanings in metaphors, expressions, figures of speech or idioms, such as, 'pull your socks up', or 'he wears his heart on his sleeve'. A striking example of this is the story of the teacher who said to the autistic pupil, 'Don't worry; your mother is going to be late; she's tied up in the office'. The little boy immediately started screaming because he thought somebody had tied his mother up. I had an interesting experience once in a therapy session with a young lady who had recently been diagnosed with autism. She had just obtained an 'Autism Alert Card', to which I said, 'That's a useful thing to have up your sleeve'. Ten minutes later she told me that she had been on the back of her boyfriend's motorbike, to which I replied, 'That sounds a bit hairy'. She was confused by the ambiguity of my expressions, later saying on reflection:

> 'I don't understand about 10% of what you or other people say, but I just nod and pretend I do. It's like people sometimes speak a different language. Writing an email is easier than talking for me. When talking I feel less in control and less fluent. Mainly I struggle to understand the words, as the true meaning of the speaker often seems to contradict the words they use'.

The autistic person is often confused by teasing, joking, irony, innuendo and sarcasm, failing to pick up on intentions or hidden meanings and having a tendency to make a literal interpretation. However, with age, come greater awareness, understanding and the development of coping skills.

Willey (1999, p23) commented,

> As a child I took language and words very literally. Metaphors, similes and analogies did not exist to me. I never considered that a statement had more than one meaning. I was continually baffled by what people said. My parents and teachers thought I was being obstinate, disobedient, audacious, and pedantic... I understood their language, knew if

they made grammatical errors in their speech, but I never understood their vernacular. I was unable to read between the lines, subtexts and innuendoes, to understand the thought processes of my peers.

A further important part of non-verbal communication in a conversation is our ability to vary intonation and volume, to emphasise certain words, in order to add emotion. Some autistic people struggle with this skill, leaving their speech with a rather flat, monotonous quality. For some people, their speech is slightly too loud, has a high-pitched or nasal quality and does not convey the social and emotional information that enriches language. Some children have had training and advice from speech and language therapists on how to improve their prosody by using the kind of techniques that actors use. Autistic people may, themselves, not only have difficulty with displaying variations in tone, and volume, but also often struggle to interpret the hidden meaning in other people's intonation. One further difficulty that mainly occurs in children is known as 'echolalia', where the child will learn phrases from other people and repeat them in exactly the same way as they've heard them.

## Language: reciprocal two-way conversations

Smooth, reciprocal conversations are often challenging for autistic people as there are all sorts of components: knowing how to start with an 'opener', building on what the other person has said, timing a comment so as not to talk over the other person, changing the topic smoothly, not jumping from topic to topic without an obvious link or reference, making 'check-out comments' such as 'Do you know what I mean?', or 'Really', or verbal and non-verbal reinforcers such as 'Hmm', 'Yes' 'Uhuh' or head nodding and knowing how to end a conversation. For many autistic people this type of reciprocal conversation doesn't come naturally or intuitively and has to become a learnt skill. Reciprocal conversation involves not only articulating one's own thoughts, but also at the same time having an awareness of what the other person is thinking, feeling and saying, responding with 'everyday and informal non-verbal behaviour' and linking it all together. This requires multiple channels of attention to be processing information at the same time. Duncan gave an insightful report into the difficulties many autistic people have, saying:

> For me my conversations don't flow smoothly like a river, I find it difficult to get into a rhythm. When I watch other people's conversation it is like a game of table tennis, with lots of backwards and forwards – I find that difficult to do. I often don't know where to start, or what to say. I will go off on tangents following my own thoughts and sometimes will talk over the other person.

Another client, Richard, had more severe difficulties, saying that as a child he really struggled with language, not speaking fluently until the age of 5. He commented,

> Thinking and speech don't go together naturally for me. I struggle to think and speak at the same time. Then if the person I'm talking to wants eye contact on top of that, it's often too much. In my mind it's a question of, 'Do you want eye contact or a conversation? I can't do both.'

Continuing the theme of single channel communication, sometimes autistic individuals are good public speakers, or actors, which I initially found surprising. I once attended a conference where I found unexpectedly that one of the clients whom I had assessed was giving a talk. She was a brilliant speaker. At coffee break, I approached her and asked about her ability, to which she said,

> I know that I am good at giving public talks on stage about my autism because I'm talking *at* people about my special interest, but I'm not very good at talking *to* people. At the coffee break I will struggle and be much more anxious standing in a group and having a backwards and forwards conversation with three or four people. My partner tells me that my conversation tends to be one way and that I tend to 'hold court' or 'go off on a monologue', which is ideal when you are on a stage, but not great in other settings.

Sometimes an autistic person may struggle to alter their language according to the social context or even appreciate the social context. For example, if somebody says, 'How are you today?' as you pass them in the corridor, the context requires a brief response with few details. In fact, it's just a way of saying hello. It's rhetorical, a trick question; the other person usually doesn't want a conversation. They may just expect you to say, 'Fine thanks and yourself?' and pass on.

For some autistic people, there is a strong desire to finish what they have started, without interruptions, irrespective of the other person's response. This can be worse if the person has poor eye contact or is unaware that the listener might not be interested. One man said, 'It is almost as if I have found somebody to listen and now have the opportunity to talk, and talk I will'.

Often the autistic person is unsure of what the other person wants, sometimes they will not take into account how much the other person knows, which results in them either providing too much detailed information or too little. The person might not be able to organise a 'narrative framework', follow a theme or clearly report an event for disclosure because they get caught up and derailed in the details, going off on tangents and missing the point of the story or the punch line.

I asked one client how he had met his wife as they seemed rather an incongruous couple, the woman was a middle-class, well-spoken, university graduate with a career and he was a man with no educational qualifications, no job or career prospects and a tendency to ramble on about obscure technical subjects. 'I met Juliet when I was fixing her car. I ended up welding the floor of her Morris Minor which was in a shocking condition – really rusty.

The camshaft had gone on …' He then spent 10 minutes describing with great enthusiasm the inside of Juliet's engine and the mechanical specifications of the Morris Minor and completely missed the point of my question which was, 'Can you explain how you two people are together and have stayed together for 10 years, when you are obviously so very different?' I did not want to know details about the car she had 10 years ago!

## Language: pedantic (too formal)

Pedantic language usually implies giving too much correct information, too much detail, but not being aware of what the other person really needs to hear. Some adults with autism may be overly formal, pedantic and over precise in their choice of language. As children their speech is often, 'too adult' or correct, and instead of saying, 'Mum said don't do that', they might say, 'My mother said I should not do that'. Being precise might mean that instead of saying, 'last summer', they might be more precise and say 'on the 27th of July last year'. One client said that when she was a child and answered the house phone, people thought she was an adult. There is an inflexibility in being pedantic, for example, not taking short cuts, having to get everything just right, not liking to be interrupted, having to finish a thought.

One man said, 'I am acutely sensitive to words and can be quite obsessive. I obsess about whether one word is better than another to express my thoughts, which takes a long time. I need my thoughts to be perfectly formed before I allow them to leave my mouth'. Another one said, 'I'm a grammar Nazi and get caught up in insignificant detail about whether people use "is" when it should be "are", "of" instead of "off", and their use of modal verbs or apostrophes really annoys me'. Liane Holliday Willey (1999) said, 'Language appeals to me because it lends itself to rules and precision' (p38).

## Types of sensory sensitivity

Nine out of ten autistic people process sensory information differently from their non-autistic peers. This might mean they find everyday sounds and textures overwhelming or have difficulty recognising pain or where their body is in space. Imagine that everything you see, taste, touch, hear and smell comes at you with the same intensity. It is difficult to filter and focus on one thing, so that environments like supermarkets and swimming pools are overwhelming and painful. Over the past few decades, clinicians have become more aware of the problem of sensory sensitivities in autistic people confirmation of this being that 'sensory issues' are now a key symptom in the diagnostic manual DSM-V. For some autistic people 'sensory sensitivity' or 'sensory integration difficulties' have a greater negative impact on their lives than problems that are created in the social and emotional world due to restricted behaviours. There are three main types of sensory processing issues in autism: (1) hyper (over) sensitive, where sensations are perceived as unbearably intense and intolerable; (2) hypo (under) sensitive, where there might be an absence of sensation or (3) mono-processing, where only one sense is processed at a time. Learning how to manage sensory issues helps one to avoid overload or 'meltdowns' and improves quality of life. The main sense areas are as follows:

- Auditory (hearing, sound, noise).

- Visual (sight, light, colour).

- Olfactory (smell).

- Tactile (touch, pain, temperature).

- Gustatory (taste, hunger).

- Vestibular (movement, balance).

- Proprioception (awareness of body in space).

Many people would grimace at the sensation of nails being scratched down a blackboard, but imagine what it would be like if your hearing was hypersensitive and that reaction occurred for you in many situations. Grandin (2006) commented,

> Loud noises hurt my ears like a dentist drill hitting a nerve … for others touch can be painful – like razors drawn across the skin … the ringing of the school bell always hurt my ears… As a baby I resisted being touched and when I became a little older, I can remember stiffening, flinching and pulling away from relatives when they hugged me.

When living with a mixture of these sensitivities, the world can become a threatening place, with the possibility of a dangerous environment around every corner. Charlotte recalled her schooldays as being a painful memory because of her sensory issues, never being quite sure where the next painful sensory experienced lurked:

> At school, the dining room, playground and corridors were a constant insult to my senses as they were so noisy, coupled with the fluorescent lights, bells ringing and people bumping into each other. Then there was the smell of different cleaning products and people's scent and perfumes. Going to school was a nightmare. I can only describe it as like being in the jungle where around every corner there was an impending danger or if you imagine what it would be like to be stuck in a giant spin drier. Afterwards I'd feel really tired or drained.

We do not have a full understanding of the roots of these difficulties, but we know it is a neurological problem concerned with the way the brain processes and analyses information from our receptive sense organs – the ears, eyes, nose, tongue, skin and stomach. Our sense organs transform sensory stimuli (light, sound, odour etc.) into electrical and chemical signals, which are identified, parcelled together and interpreted by the brain. Many autistic people have difficulty processing sensory input for more than one sense at a time. The term often used to describe this is 'monotropic', or single channelled, which means struggling to process more than one channel simultaneously. This appears most common in the auditory and visual pathways and may explain why some individuals struggle to look at other people when they are having a conversation. Fay said, 'When I was a child, people would say, "Look at me when I'm talking to you", but I found it distracting and it overloaded my senses. My ideal position to talk to somebody would be sitting back to back or sitting alongside somebody who is in the passenger seat of a car'.

A further problem is the inability to filter out and ignore background information, and to focus on foreground information. One man recently commented, 'I found it really difficult having a conversation with my mother in her flat because I could hear, and was distracted by, the sound of the neighbours through the thin walls next door'. Often autistic people report feeling bombarded with information from simultaneous sources and are vulnerable to sensory overload. Tina commented,

> A shopping centre or an airport sends me into sensory overdrive - the noise, the lights, its intensity, flashing and stuffiness. I cope by walking (very) swiftly through the duty free, breathing through my mouth with head down and headphones on.

## Sensory sensitivities: hearing, sight, touch, taste and smell

*Hearing and sounds:* the most common sensory sensitivity is to hearing, which might include any combination of the following: (1) distress caused by a sudden unexpected noise like a dog barking, an alarm going off, a bell or a balloon bursting or high-pitched continuous noises, for example, from an electric motor or vacuum cleaner; (2) distress caused by confusing, mixed, overlapping noises such as the cacophony in a shopping centre, busy restaurant or a school playground – unable to hear one voice among others; (3) distress caused by hearing noise that other people don't notice such as a ticking clock or the sound of the central heating. On a more positive note, some people on the autism spectrum are so sensitive to sound and differentiating sounds that they have 'perfect pitch' and become expert musicians. See Table 5.2 Sensory issues and coping strategies.

*Sight and light:* sensitivity to bright lights, such as midday sunlight or particular types of lighting such as a fluorescent lights or flickering light, or the overwhelming visual stimulation in a supermarket, can be troubling. One man said he was 'blinded by brightness', which was why he wore sunglasses. Occasionally, there might be sensitivity to a particular colour; one woman said that she couldn't stand anything that was red. Sometimes there might be poor depth perception which results in difficulties throwing or catching a ball. There can also be an intense fascination with certain visual details such as noticing a pattern on a carpet or a tiny scrap of paper on a floor. That super sensitivity to detail and pattern can result in the artistic and technical ability to copy an image accurately in fine detail.

*Touch and textures:* sensitivity to certain scratchy textures, such as wool, labels on clothes or the seams in socks are common issues. Many autistic people dislike being touched, or more particularly, they find the deep pressure of being squeezed more bearable than a light unexpected touch. Deborah Lipsky, is autistic writes in her book *From Anxiety to Meltdown* (2011) of the similarity between some autistic people and herd animals, such as deer, cattle and horses – she owns an animal rescue centre. Lipsky notes that herd animals have hypervigilant senses, a startle response to light touch and an aversion to direct eye contact. For example, a horse touched very lightly will tend to react with a startle and perceive direct eye contact to be threatening. Lipsky suggests that this is why autistic people might communicate and bond so well with animals.

*Smell:* some people on the spectrum have very strong likes and dislikes for certain smells, finding certain aromas overpowering and intense. Common disliked smells include perfumes, deodorants, scents, chemicals in paints and disinfectants. On the positive side, one client's sensitivity to smell and the accuracy with which she could differentiate smell helped her greatly in developing a career as a perfume maker. Another client, Paulo, a successful Italian IT consultant, told the story of how his sensory difficulties with smell created problems for his love life:

> On one occasion a girl turned up for a date reeking of really strong perfume. I just had to say, 'Your smell is really too strong, could you please have a shower before we start talking, otherwise I will not be able to concentrate for the whole evening'. She wasn't very happy but complied and we had a nice evening.

However, one client built a career, based on his highly sensitive sense of smell and taste, as a specialist wine taster. His job involved authenticating and differentiating between very expensive old wines. Another client worked as a perfumer, saying that, 'I hold in my memory a big library of smells, some from 25 years ago. I go around the world looking for flowers with new smells to add to my company's cosmetics range'.

*Taste and texture:* sensitivity to taste and texture of food is also fairly common in people on the spectrum and often results in people becoming rather fussy eaters. Jake's comment below is fairly typical:

> I can't have foods mixed up on a plate and I can't stand food being covered with a sauce. I eat each food separately. Why would you want to mix the taste of a carrot with meat? I am also supersensitive

to anything that has a slimy texture and prefer food that is dry and, for example, always eat my cereal dry without milk.

Many autistic adults have quite a restricted diet, often getting into a routine of eating the same food for breakfast, lunch and dinner. As long as

*Table 5.2* Sensory issues and coping strategies

| Sensory issues | Coping strategy |
| --- | --- |
| **Hearing and sound** | |
| Hard to focus on what somebody is saying – distracted by other low-level noises like a ticking clock, fan or light buzzing. | Turn off or remove background noise if possible. Go to a quiet place when you really need to focus. Use headphones to block out background noise. |
| Find loud noises (bells, alarms, hoovers, hand driers) bothersome and even painful. | Use noise-cancelling earplugs which allow you to hear pertinent information but reduce the overall noise level. |
| Hear things that others don't notice, e.g. clocks, neighbours. | Either remove the stimulus or try to mask it with calming repetitive sounds or music. |
| **Sight and light** | |
| Difficulty tolerating lighting such as fluorescent lights or bright sunlight. | Change lighting, use lamps or low-watt bulbs or take breaks. Wear dark glasses or a hat with a brim. |
| Find places with a great deal of visual information overwhelming (e.g. supermarkets). | Avoid large busy stores, or shop at quieter times. Take your glasses off so you can't see as clearly or wear sunglasses. |
| Disorientated or unable to relax in certain decorative environments. | Create calming spaces with limited visual input in your home. Have blank walls if necessary. |
| Unable to find items in a busy environment. | Create systems, use filing cabinets and labels so things stand out. |
| **Touch** | |
| Certain clothes or labels are unpleasant and I struggle to ignore the irritation. | Choose soft clothes and bed sheets. Cut out the labels. Wear an undervest. |
| Finds light touch from others particularly troubling. | Inform that you don't like it and that you would prefer deep pressure or a squeeze. |
| Finds unplanned touch and hugs stressful. | Ask the person to tell you when the touch is starting and finishing. |
| Finds personal grooming activities such as shaving, brushing teeth or cutting hair difficult. | Try different hairdressers, shaving kits or toothbrushes until you find the least noxious. |
| Strong dislike of being too hot or cold. | Be more aware of your environment and choice of clothing. |
| **Smell** | |
| Finds certain smells or someone wearing perfume or aftershave upsetting. | Breathe in through your mouth rather than nose. Carry an alternative favourite smell on a scarf or tissue that is soothing. Let people know you have a smell sensitivity. |
| Wearing perfume gives me a headache. Aversion to some cleaning and bathing products. | Don't wear perfume. Buy non-scented cleaning and bathing products. |
| **Taste** | |
| Strong dislike of various tastes and texture of food. | Try to strike a balance between following your preferences, expanding your range and mixing similar foods. |
| Dislike of slimy food. | Try mixing up slimy sensations by adding crunchy food such as celery or nuts. |

the person has the right nutritional ingredients, this might not be a problem. But this is an area where people can attempt to be more flexible in a graduated way, trying to systematically desensitise themselves to different and varied foods. This desensitisation approach means very gradually, in stages, trying to expose themselves to an aversive food, initially just touching it, then maybe licking it and finally maybe putting it in their mouth and swallowing it.

## Other sensitivities to bodily states: temperature, pain, hunger

Occasionally, a person will have a lack of sensitivity or awareness of bodily states such as hunger. One mother said, 'I didn't realise Ellie didn't know when she was hungry or not until one day when she was about six years old, I said "Are you hungry?" to which she replied, "How would I know?" In Ellie's situation, there is a lack of connectivity between the appetite centre in the brain and the frontal thinking awareness part of the brain, and so the message that the body was hungry simply didn't get through. A similar lack of connectivity might occur in other situations, for example when the child isn't aware of being cold or in pain. Some people have very high tolerance of pain and are not aware of life-threatening injuries or illnesses, which may result in putting themselves into risky situations or having to make more frequent trips to the hospital. Having to cope with these extreme sensory experiences means autistic people sometimes appear very stoical, not flinching or showing distress, in response to pain that others would consider unbearable. This characteristic is a useful trait for people who engage in extreme endurance sports, such as long-distance running or cycling, or even services in the military where tolerance of extreme discomfort is a prerequisite. But if these signals that alert the person to danger are absent, they might be more prone to long-term injury.

## Sensory overload, meltdowns and coping

An accumulation of sensory stresses, combined with other life's stresses, including stress associated with socialising, can sometimes lead to overload and 'meltdowns'. Tamzin commented,

> I flipped, flew into a rage the moment my sensory system became overloaded. I call it 'brain fuzz', like a television being on the blink. I was already stressed at work. On top of that I've always hated fluorescent lights. I was wearing a skirt I didn't really like and new shoes which were uncomfortable. But what tipped me over the edge was when the fire alarm went off. It was only a fire practice but it was just the final straw.

Temple Grandin invented a hug or squeeze machine after realising that deep pressure can reduce her hypersensitivity and the anxiety it causes. The idea for this device came when she noticed that the cattle being branded in a squeeze chute at her aunt's farm calmed down as soon as the pressure was administered. Grandin built a machine for herself which could vary the pressure and time duration of the squeeze depending on her own needs. Willey (2008, p30) described having 'safety zones' where she could get away from sensory overload, such as climbing into an alcove under her bed:

> Whenever things became too fuzzy, or loud or too distracting; whenever I began to feel as though I would become unravelled, I knew I could crawl into my alcove and crunch up into it, until I felt a square and symmetry. I could squeeze my knees and pull my thoughts back into my bones.

Sometimes people find it best to explain their difficulties to others. Stephen found that by telling people he had 'sensory integration problems', it helped explain his poor eye contact: 'I find it useful to say to people, "I just want you to know that although I'm looking down at the floor, I'm hearing every word you say". I have visual and auditory sensory integration difficulties that make sustaining eye contact difficult'.

Some sensitivities diminish with age but generally it is a lifelong condition. However, some of the techniques listed next can help:

(a) *Be aware of sensory issues:* the most important step in coping is becoming more aware of your own sensory issues and how it affects you.

(b) *Be your own advocate and learn to take care of yourself:* be assertive and give yourself permission to accept your sensory sensitivities.

(c) *Explain to others such as friends and family about sensory sensitivities:* tell people what the issues are and seek their understanding.

(d) *Avoidance of the stimuli and modification of the environment is often best:* avoidance and modification may be necessary. For example, ask for a quiet table in a restaurant, or ask for the music to be turned down.

(e) *Carry a portable sensory first aid kit:* including items such as sunglasses, ear plugs, a pleasant scent, a book, music or a favourite tactile object.

(f) *Systematic desensitisation:* this tool doesn't seem effective with autism-type sensory sensitivities as there appears to be no habituation or decrease in anxiety on exposure.

(g) *Self-talk can help:* with maturity, endurance/tolerance can increase. Self-talk for example saying, 'This won't last long; I'll be out of here in 10 minutes', can help.

(h) *Script:* consider having a pre-prepared script that you can show others at times when you need help but find it difficult to communicate.

    i *Be practical, control and diminish discomfort:* control the things that you can control, so when the unexpected occurs, you are not already stressed. For example, wear clothes that are comfortable.

    ii *Make your home a sensory-safe comfort base:* when facing sensory challenges in the outside world, have a safe, comfortable place to retreat back to.

## Synaesthesia and creative thought

Synaesthesia, literally meaning, 'union of the senses', is a complex sensory phenomenon where there is a blending of sensation, perception and emotion – the senses get mixed up. Around 2–4% of the general population have a degree of synaesthesia, but around 20% of autistic people have the condition. The most common type is where a person might see numbers as colours; for example number three is seen as blue. But other people report experiencing other phenomena; a taste when listening to music, tasting a colour, seeing a sound, hearing a shape, seeing faces with coloured halos or emotions provoking a certain colour. The condition is thought to be because of an anomaly in the wiring (connectivity) of the brain, where there is cross wiring or cross activation. It is no coincidence that the main colour recognition area of the brain is the fusiform gyrus of the temporal lobe, which is the same general area that specialises in number and face recognition. It could be that the wiring for number has mistakenly been put in the neighbouring connection for colour, so that the person sees colour for numbers.

There is evidence that synaesthesia is particularly linked to savant abilities and sensory sensitivities in autism rather than autism per se. Ramachandra (2011) points out that as well as mathematicians, many creative artists, writers, musicians, painters and poets – Kandinsky, Pollock, Nabakov, Liszt – had or have synaesthesia, and he estimates that one-sixth of all creative people have the condition. His research also suggests that synaesthesia has a genetic component and runs in families. It is often the ability to forge links between seemingly unrelated domains of the brain, linking unrelated words, images and ideas that are the core of creativity. A poet or writer who creates a metaphor is in a sense creating a link between two domains, linking seemingly unrelated concepts, words, images and ideas. Our ability to uncover hidden analogies is the basis of creative thought. Shakespeare was particularly good at creating metaphors and imagery – one of my favourites is, 'Friends, grapple them to the soul, with hoops of steel'. There must have been a good connection, a bundle of long white neural fibres, between Shakespeare's vocabulary or word part of his brain and the visual-spatial pictorial areas.

Two creative autistic clients, first Jenny a writer and Gordon a musician commented,

- My sensory experiences are unusual, but I wouldn't change them. Okay, my hearing which is over sensitive to noise is really annoying and stressful and I would change that. But, I think I gain so much beauty and meaning from how my senses work. I do see and note colour in people's voices, I sometimes get a strong taste of lemon with particular people, I get tactile feelings particularly on my skin with music and certain words make me feel warm. I think it all helps my creativity.

- I'm now a Professor of Music and I'm aware that I have a sensory ability that I'm disappointed that most of my students don't have. When I hear a piece of music I can visualise the notes as a sequence of numbers and literally digitalise the music. For some reason I've been able to do this from childhood.

## Motor coordination and body awareness

It is estimated that 80% of autistic people have problems with motor coordination, body awareness (proprioception) or clumsiness. The first indicators are often difficulties learning to walk, which might be delayed by a few months. As they grow older, children might also show difficulties learning to dress, tie up shoelaces, use a knife, fork, scissors, do up buttons, knot a neck tie or learn to skate. They might also show clumsiness or have a tendency to bump into things. They might have an odd gait when running or walking and an ungainly lack of coordination and synchronicity between upper and lower limbs. Others might have difficulty catching or throwing a ball, which is to do with timing and poor coordination. Some children walk without the associated arm swing or have a problem with balance and therefore find riding a bicycle very difficult; others might have a problem clapping in rhythm. Poor handwriting is a common problem and is part of the dyspraxic area of difficulty associated with poor movement and fine motor coordination or bilateral coordination problems.

People on the autism spectrum are often not very good at team sports that require fine coordination, although many have become good at solitary sport such as long-distance running, where a low tolerance for discomfort is an advantage, or individual sports such as golf, swimming, rock climbing, archery, horse riding or martial arts. Receiving a separate diagnosis of dyspraxia, from autism, is common. Others might have involuntary tics (motor or verbal) or facial twitches as in Tourette's syndrome. As stated in Chapter 2, the part of the brain called the cerebellum – concerned with the calibration, integration and coordination of fine motor movement, dexterity and timing – is smaller in a high proportion of autistic people, which might explain the difficulties expressed next:

- I never had a sense of natural grace; it was as if my brain and body were not connected properly. When I played football at school, my feet would get all tangled up and I'd often miss the ball.

- The pencil did not obey me; it just felt awkward in my hand.

- I always felt disconnected between my body and my brain and really struggle to keep in time with a rhythm if people are clapping to music.

- Sometimes my shadow is my best friend because it shows me what I'm doing. I don't have a sense of my body in space.

On a positive note, Amanda initially trained as a dancer and had what is described as, 'superior visual motor discrimination' and became a very successful dance notary. This is the person who writes movement scores for dance sequences and choreography, using graphic symbols, figures and letters, in the same way that a musician would write down the musical sequences in terms of notes on a score sheet. Amanda can watch a sequence of movements, hold it in mind, then write down on paper the symbols required to reconstruct that sequence of movements in the future.

This chapter demonstrates the range of impact of the condition, the diversity of the client group and the pervasive nature of these difficulties. Autism can produce extremes, super memory, exceptional mathematical abilities, an eye for language, an eye for the details of life, heightened sensitivities to sound, vision, taste, smell and touch and even an ability to focus intensely and endure discomfort. The flip side is that it might bring with it an embarrassing forgetfulness for faces, poor multitasking ability, slowed processing speed, problems reading a map, poor handwriting and intolerance of certain noises and textures. This great diversity of characteristics that blend together differently, not only adds to life's rich tapestry, but also brings to mind the popular saying, first mentioned in chapter One that, it is difficult to make generalizations and that 'If you've met one person with autism, you've met one person with autism' (Shore, 2006).

# CHAPTER 6

# Emotions and the social and relational world

## Emotions – interoception and introspection

Do you ever wonder if you experience emotions too intensely or not intensely enough? Have you got the balance right between thinking and feeling – mind and heart? Some autistic people struggle with understanding and processing emotions, and their experience can be a mirror to help us all understand ourselves more fully. One autistic client said to me once, 'How can I understand the emotions in another person if I can't understand the emotions in myself?' Our understanding and experience of our own feelings is due to a combination of factors: (1) the relational or emotional environment we were brought up in (nurture) and (2) the wiring or connectivity of our brain (nature).

First, let's start off with 'nurture' and a brief summary of child development research over the last 80 years. In essence, we know that being raised in a loving, caring environment, where adults form emotional attachments and respond contingently, in synchrony with the infant, reinforcing and shaping emotional responses, provides an optimal environment to grow up in. On the other hand, emotional deprivation, abuse, trauma and invalidation are not good for healthy emotional development. The infant needs a supportive environment where they are allowed to experience and label a range of emotions. With appropriate guidance, rules and boundaries, the infant gradually learns to regulate their emotions. Parents of autistic children are no different to anybody else in terms of these parenting skills. However, an undiagnosed autistic child might pose a few more challenges as they might not be 'tuned in' to the neurotypical world, or the neurotypical parents might not be 'tuned in' to the autistic world; therefore, this synchronised emotional and behavioural responding is more difficult to achieve.

Second, let's look at 'nature', with the implication that we are born with individual differences, different genes, different wiring and connectivity in our brains. Research studies Garfinkel et al, 2016; Fiene and Brownlow, 2015) suggest that autistic people are poorer at 'interoception' or 'the awareness or noting of changes in bodily sensations', which might be bodily signals for hunger, thirst, pain, fear, a tickle, sexual arousal or rapid heartbeat. If the sensation is not noticed, it is more difficult to label or name it and interpret it as an emotion. So, for example, an autistic person, with this poor connectivity might not automatically realise, 'My heart is beating quickly, my muscles are tense, I am sweating, therefore I must be anxious or frightened'. One suggestion for this phenomenon is that the insula cortex, a key relay station on the pathway between our sensory brain and frontal lobes, is less active in autistic individuals (Nomi et al, 2019) (see Chapter 2, Figure 6.1). The insula is folded deep within the fissure between the frontal and temporal lobes and its job is to receive signals from all the visceral organs in the body, such as the heart, lungs, liver, bones, muscles and skin. It then forms a map of the sensations that are being experienced in the different parts of the body. The insula then passes on the information, for example, 'My heart is beating quickly; I must be anxious or excited'. If the person doesn't get those messages clearly and lacks awareness of bodily sensations that reflect emotions, they can be in effect, blind or deaf to their own bodily sensations or states, including emotions. One client, Emily, commented, 'I've always had a hard time pinpointing my symptoms when I'm not feeling very well. I also don't know if I'm hungry and I don't get that signal that says, "You are thirsty and need a drink". Similarly, I don't know if I'm stressed, anxious or angry until I'm completely overwhelmed'.

Often autistic people report that they need to deliberately monitor and scan their body, checking it out with an emotional thermometer, to get a clue as to how they are feeling. The better connected a brain, the smoother the transmission, backwards and forwards, between sensation, thought and feelings. Grandin (2006, p40) said, 'My brain scan showed that emotional circuits between my frontal cortex and the amygdala just aren't hooked up – circuits that affect my emotions and are tied to my ability to love'.

**Body State**
The urge to act when thirsty

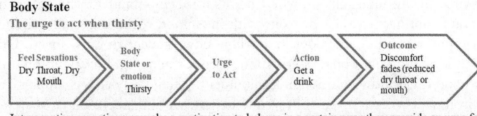

Interoceptive sensations provoke a motivation to behave in a certain way; they provide an urge for an action.

**Emotional State**
The urge to act when frustrated

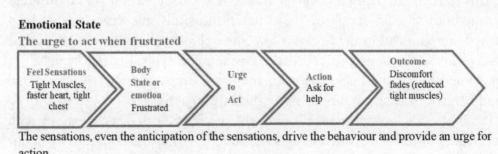

The sensations, even the anticipation of the sensations, drive the behaviour and provide an urge for action.

*Figure 6.1* Similarity between body/sensory state and emotional state (Adapted from Mahler, 2015)

There is a further level of emotional awareness, called 'introspection', which is the ability to stand back and reflect on our own thoughts, feelings and responses. For example, I might think, 'I'm getting anxious, I can feel my heart thumping because I've got to give a speech in front of all those people: I'm slightly worried I'm not fully prepared. I'll take 15 minutes to look at my notes'. This level of 'introspection' involves reflecting on inner experiences, using words to make connections and particularly identifying external triggers and ways of reacting. This requires a level of abstract thought as emotions and feelings are in themselves abstract concepts. Sometimes an autistic people might tend to have a rather 'black and white' literal view and might have difficulty recognising abstract concepts such as emotions, which are not as easily understood as the logical, rational world associated with numbers, rules, structures and systems.

## Possible differences in the way autistic people process emotions

### Time delay

There is evidence of a slower speed of information processing and reduced efficiency in switching attentional channels on the autism spectrum. To explain slower emotional processing, Temple Grandin uses the metaphor of autistic people having a 'dialup' rather than 'high-speed' Internet connection'. Some clients have made the following comments:

- 'It takes a while for the emotion to percolate through. It's like my timing is different and I'm on a time delay. I cope with the facts first, then the emotions take over so I'm not overloaded. I don't process things as smoothly. Sometimes I store things up and then explode or have a meltdown – it's all or nothing'.

- 'I've always had a strong emotional disconnect. I get it on a cognitive level but not on a feeling level. There might be a three-day delay'.

- 'My strongest emotional reactions are often delayed and it took me almost a month to cry after my grandmother's funeral'.

- 'When I got the diagnosis, the psychologist said, "How does that make you feel?" I didn't feel anything; I knew I needed time to process it. Now I feel very happy about it'.

### Different degrees or range of emotion – smaller wavelength

Tony Attwood expounds the view that generally autistic people experience a smaller band or wavelength of emotional responses – almost hypoemotional, experiencing a general lower level of emotions. They are not so jolly and happy at Christmas or celebrations, not so excited about going on exotic holidays and not so sad at funerals or tragedies. Temple Grandin explains, 'My emotions are all in the present. I can be angry, but I get over it quickly. When I replay a scene, the emotions are no longer attached to them'. Grandin goes on to say that, 'I am what I do, not what I feel' and says she doesn't get complex lingering emotions. An autistic person might approach emotions in a logical way with more thinking than feeling. Other people on the spectrum report greater extremes of emotion, experiencing peaks and spikes (hyperemotionality) as with other senses, but these emotions don't linger or last for long. People have made the following comments:

- 'There are advantages to being unemotional. My girlfriend said she liked me because I was always calm, steady and "like a rock", in a crisis. I'm very logical and just think things through. I think I'd be a very good doctor in A&E'.

- 'At my grandmother's funeral I pretended I was sad like everybody else and had to restrain myself from being silly and trying to cheer everybody up'.

- 'I'm "aemotional", if that is a word – I'm not happy or sad. I'm just here. Sometimes I do have emotional responses; sometimes I don't; sometimes I don't know. Most of the time I'm just OK'.

- 'I won an award at work for my database and had to go to an award ceremony. Everybody was getting excited and slapping me on the back, but I felt a bit of a killjoy because I just thought, "So what, I was just doing my job"'.

- 'If I go into a shop, I never choose anything spontaneously. I've never had that "gut reaction". All my decisions are based on logical appraisal'.

- 'I find it difficult to resonate with the happiness of others'.

- 'When my dog died, I did cry and was sad for a couple of hours, but it passed and my rational mind kicked back in. My wife has been upset for the last two months'.

## All or nothing emotions – switching on and off

Closely linked to not feeling certain emotions is the notion that for many people with an autism diagnosis, their is a tendency to be either black (bad, negative) or white (good, happy neutral) – 'all or nothing' – with no shades of grey, nothing in the middle. People have made the following comments:

- 'My mind doesn't realise it's feeling something until the very last minute; then it's very extreme. Now I'm beginning to recognise more when I'm feeling emotion – particularly since I got my diagnosis and I'm seeing a therapist. I notice my breathing is becoming quicker and I get a bit shaky if I'm becoming anxious. If there are tears behind my eyes, I'm feeling sad, or the sandbag on top of my heart is lifted when I feel relaxed. I now make a list, a sort of diary and connect things up in my mind. I don't pick up internal bodily messages very well so I can't tell if I'm hungry, or if my bladder is full, until the very last minute. It's the same with feeling stressed – it's rather black and white like a switch – all or nothing!'

- 'To me life is "happy" or "not happy", "angry" or "not angry". I don't tend to feel the in-between emotions, it's either one or the other'.

- 'My therapist gave me an Emotional Colour Wheel and a diagram of an Emotional Thermometer, which were very useful tools that were very helpful in identifying and grading my emotions'. (see page 203)

## Somatisation – emotion expressed physically

When we are stressed, there are often physical manifestations of that stress – we might be more prone to a cold, headache or diarrhoea – but often people on the autism spectrum lack that awareness of the emotion of stress and just see the physical manifestation. For some, the physical manifestation might 'come out of the blue'.

- 'Before I got my diagnosis if somebody had said to me, "Do you have anxiety?" I'd have said, "No". But I did have this thing called "unexplained nausea", where I would vomit and then feel physically drained. I've since realised that was my anxiety – that was how my body expressed it; I just wasn't good at sensing it'.

- 'I lost my job and although I knew I was upset, for three days I just felt dizzy and sick'.

- 'Every time I went to see my therapist, I got a pain in my face and aches in my neck and back because I was so tense; my neck muscles are now visibly stronger. In the past I would never have agreed that I had anxiety or stress'.

## Discomfort and other reactions to strong emotion in others

Many autistic individuals are uncomfortable with prolonged high emotional intensity in others, possibly due to not having those feelings themselves and thus being unequipped to interpret and respond. Other people on the spectrum report that they do pick up on other people's strong emotions, but it is sometimes not a conscious, cognitive process, but almost a sensing, an intuitive feeling, sometimes described as being like a 'contagion' or catching the emotion from somebody else.

- 'Emotions of others make me feel uncomfortable. They seem exaggerated, gushing and overly demonstrative'.

- 'I find emotional weakness and neediness in other people very tiring – I really find it difficult to tolerate'.

- 'Expressing emotions is difficult. Females are often all huggy and kissy, which is not my cup of tea. I can feel something quite profound inside, but it doesn't always show on my face'.

- 'My first boyfriend was all over me like a rash. He'd always want to touch, hold hands and tell me he loved me – it drove me mad. He had to go. My husband is much cooler and unemotional which suits me better'.

- 'I pick up other people's moods subconsciously. If someone approaches me for a conversation and is full of fear and anger, I find myself suddenly in that same state of emotion'. (See Appendix 1 page 203)

## Alexithymia or 'emotional literacy' – lack of words for emotions

Alexithymia is a term coined to describe a state of deficiency in understanding, processing or describing emotions; it literally means, 'without words for mood or emotions'. It is the inverse of concepts such as 'psychological mindedness', 'emotional intelligence' and 'introspection'. It involves difficulty identifying feelings and distinguishing between feelings and bodily sensations and being unable to describe feelings to other people. Alexithymia is thought to be greater in males than females and occurs in less than 10% of the general population (although over 50% of the autistic population). The answer to the question 'How are you feeling?' is often very more difficult for the autistic person as they may not actually fully know and don't have the words to provide an answer.

- 'I find it hard to explain how I feel. I don't know how to grasp mentally the intangible emotions swirling in my mind, to identify and label them and then accurately communicate those feelings in speech'.

- 'I know how to think but am not sure I know how to feel'.

- 'I find it hard to identify my emotions. The other day I was upset and it helped listening to my music, a prepared stream of pop songs. One sad song came on and I said, "That's exactly how I feel"'.

- 'Sometimes I feel my emotions in colours rather than words. I need a language for my worries'.

## Understanding and recognising emotion in others

This skill involves being able to read the emotional expression of another person, mainly through interpreting facial expression, voice intonation and non-verbal body language. This is largely a cognitive skill but also involves having a shared referent of understanding, being able to identify those same emotions in themselves.

- 'Animals I understand, people I don't. At least animals are honest. If an animal doesn't like you, it growls. If a person doesn't like you, they might smile'.

- 'I can work out what's going on emotionally, but it's not intuitive or natural. I work it out like a mathematical puzzle; it's all logic'.

- 'If you don't signpost emotions, I just don't pick them up. I don't do non-verbals. There is no point hinting. You might as well just say it'.

- 'Because things don't have an emotional impact on me, I assume they don't have an impact on others. I assume that people just want the facts but I'm beginning to realise that this is not always right. If I have a disagreement with my wife, I try to emphasise the facts and the mistakes the facts were causing – a simple fact check could spare wounded feelings and everybody would be happier. She said my search for accuracy and quest for facts was not helpful and was irritating and I needed to focus on her hurt. She said, "Hurt feelings don't respond to your facts"'.

- 'At the end of the assessment session, when the psychologist said that I had autism, I noticed that Mum started crying. I couldn't understand why. Later she told me that she was crying out of relief and joy that after living with me and my struggles for 25 years, someone had at last identified what the key issue was'.

## Empathy

Empathy is our ability to identify what someone else is thinking and feeling and to respond to their thoughts and feelings appropriately. I would suggest that empathy can be divided into three components: cognitive empathy (knowing); emotional empathy (feeling) and compassionate empathy (responding).

Cognitive empathy (knowing) is the capacity to comprehend or read another person's point of view and is largely identified with an area of the frontal lobes called the orbitofrontal cortex. It involves the ability to read body language, facial expressions, tone of voice and other non-verbal behaviour, in order to understand the degree of distress of another person. If the emotional signals are obvious, such as the person is crying, it is relatively easy to read that emotion, rather like reading the headlines in a newspaper. But if the emotion is subtle, it is more difficult to read, like reading the small print of the article. For most autistic people, the cognitive aspects of empathy are less efficient.

Emotional or affective empathy (feeling) is the ability to experience vicariously the emotion of another person, to feel someone else's distress and to resonate with and absorb it, 'I feel what you feel', sometimes called, 'emotional contagion' or 'emotional mirroring'. It is the ability to be able to 'put yourself in someone else's shoes'. If a person with autism has never experienced those emotions, they have no emotional memory to remember back, no personal experience of that emotional depth and therefore they may have difficulty achieving empathy. However, many autistic people have very good affective or emotional empathy once they have identified the other person's distress. Sometimes autistic people are overly sensitive to another person's mood, and there can be a sensory tuning into the other person. Sharon commented, 'I have an instant subconscious reaction to the mood of others, particularly negative moods. If someone approached me full of worry or even anger, I find myself suddenly in the same state. It's almost as if my thinking ability is bypassed, I just sense it'.

Compassionate empathy (responding) is the ability to know how to respond to somebody feeling distressed in a sympathetic and appropriate manner. There is often a fear of making a mistake or being rejected when deciding how to respond and with what intensity. People on the autism spectrum might have their own reaction to distress, they might prefer to be left alone and can be awkward at providing conventional words and gestures of compassion towards other people.

Empathy requires a double-minded focus of attention, to be able to attend to both ourselves and the other person. When empathy is reduced, we become single minded or self-focused, losing sight of the other person. The following comments give a flavour of what some clients on the spectrum say about empathy:

- 'One of my colleagues, whom I managed, had a sudden death in the family and was very upset. I did what I had seen people do in films and touched her on the shoulder and said, "You go home; don't worry about anything here at work". I think I managed the situation quite well, but it was a bit like I was acting in a film'.

- 'If someone's upset, I prefer offering practical help such as making them a cup of tea, getting tissues or giving solutions – I'm not really a hugger'.

- 'I can sense or pick up feelings from others, particularly negative vibes'.

- 'Empathy doesn't come naturally to me, I'm aware I don't find it easy to take another person's perspective'.

- 'Once I notice someone has got a problem, I put myself in their shoes and, to some extent, feel just like them. This makes me feel overwhelmed and I lose sight of who I am'.

- 'I have a tendency to take on another person's emotion without realising that its not mine. Someone said it was called "Echoemotica"'.

- 'I'm a nurse on the Intensive Care Unit and I've learnt to say to parents, "I'm really sorry your baby died". But actually, I don't feel really sorry'.

- 'I've learnt to say, "I'm sorry I don't know what you are feeling but I do care"'.

- 'If there are three steps involved in empathy, I miss out on them all. I don't intuitively notice; I don't really feel or care; and I don't act'.

## Love and jealousy

It is probably true to say that generally most people on the autism spectrum are more comfortable with brief, low-intensity expressions of affection and limited tolerance of sentimentality in others and can feel overwhelmed with greater levels of expressive affection. However, at the other extreme, some autistic people can have very intense obsessive emotional reactions.

One young man called Andrew commented, 'I find it difficult to say, "I love you" to my family. When I was a child and I had to write birthday or Christmas cards for my family, I never put kisses or signed it "Love Andrew" – that would have felt wrong'. A similar honest comment was made by Rachel, in her mid-30s:

> I will never understand love; it doesn't make sense to me. I understand fear and anger; they are tangible real emotions, but love is just too abstract. I understand that I can physically fancy somebody, I know when I enjoy talking to them, or when I like them, but how do you know when you love somebody?

Both Andrew and Rachel have very logical, precise minds which perhaps do not allow them to use the word 'love' carelessly. Perhaps the word 'love' is overused today in broader society? Autistic people might wonder why non-autistic people are so obsessed with being told they are loved. The word 'love' as a concept is huge and covers a multitude of different feelings and has many implications. Indeed, it may be asked if it is the rather precise, pedantic use of language, or the lack of actual feelings, that holds Andrew and Rachel back from using the word love – or a combination of both? The ancient Greeks had at least four different words for love: *agape* – unconditional love of God and family; *eros* – erotic, sensuous love; *philia* – friendship, affection and *storge* – an empathic bond or fondness. Perhaps Andrew would be more comfortable if the definition of love was more precise, he could have said, 'I feel agape love for you, Mum'.

At the other extreme, Jade was prone to developing whirlwind attachments and infatuations, with such intensity and focus, that everything else in life was swept away. She commented,

> It was awful, I was completely obsessed with him and kept contacting him. It was so all consuming. There was no moderation – it was all or nothing. I felt like the mythical Greek character Icarus, flying into the sun. I knew my wings would burn and I'd come crashing to the ground, but I just couldn't stop myself. I know my behaviour drove him away and I was devastated.

Autistic people might not be overly physically demonstrative partners – wanting to hold hands and cuddle, but they are usually caring, loyal and affectionate, engendering a feeling of love in others. Partners of autistic people and colleagues have made the following comments:

- 'My husband is not affectionate, but he does do a lot for me – he earns the money, looks after the house – and I know his deeds show that he does love me but he has difficulty saying it'.

- 'I love Jane because she's different, loyal, and above all honest. But, at times I do feel lonely and empty, because I know she can't tap into my needs'.

- 'My husband rarely tells me he loves me. He told me once: "Look, nothing has changed; I told you when we got married that I love you". I said, "Yes, but that was five years ago!"'

- 'I was a teacher support worker for a young man with autism at university for two years and saw him most days. On my final day I really wanted him to ask me about myself or say, "How are you today?" but he didn't. I know I shouldn't have expected anything, but I did feel disappointed'.

The experience of jealousy is a complex emotion that can also illustrate something about the emotions of autistic people. I saw a couple once; the husband with autism had upset his neurotypical wife by being 'overfriendly' and slightly inappropriate with another woman at a barbeque. The wife felt jealous, saying to her husband, 'Didn't you see how she was coming on to you, flirting with you, and how you were encouraging her, laughing and joking and standing too close'. The husband did not interpret the event in the same way and could not understand the emotion of jealousy. He said, 'Why on earth would you feel like that? It doesn't make sense', which the wife felt as very dismissive. The husband was logical, not at all emotional, and prided himself on never feeling worry, doubt or negative emotions such as jealousy – he was rather intolerant of his wife's emotions calling them irrational and childish. The wife was more emotional and worried, experiencing jealousy. The husband went on to say:

> I don't feel jealous, never have and don't understand it. To me it is completely irrational. I told my wife that I love her, we have a son, so what more does she want to know? She asked me how I would feel if we were to separate and I said I would be very sad but that it would not be the end of the world. If she wanted to go off with somebody else, I wouldn't stop her – I don't want to control her. I would try to detach, unhook myself and try to put the loss aside. She said she felt devastated that I felt so little and that I was so dismissive. How she is feeling just doesn't make sense to me.

Just to prove how diverse the autism population is, Katherine, a lady in her mid-30s recently diagnosed with autism, described her experience of jealousy: 'I know what jealousy is as I've always been jealous of my younger brother. From the day he was born I didn't want him as he took my parents' attention away from me. I never referred to him by his real name, but always called him "boy" and either deliberately ignored him or was unpleasant to him'.

## Ways of improving emotional attunement

*Emotional attunement training*: children diagnosed early with autism sometimes get the opportunity to engage in 'affective or emotional education', where they can learn about the world of emotions, just as one might learn a foreign language. These special training programmes are devoted to learning how to read emotions in themselves and others. Other programmes include using comic strip stories, where the autistic person is supported to identify intentions, how others may feel and what they may be thinking, by filling in speech and thought bubbles.

*Psychotherapy/cognitive behavioural therapy*: psychological therapy is about helping people make links and connections between situations, feelings and thoughts and to self-reflect. It is advantageous if the therapist knows about autism and is directive and pragmatic, focusing on working out practical solutions and offering structured sessions.

*Learning through imitation*: many autistic people say that they deliberately read or watch TV to learn about empathic responses.

- 'I've watched hundreds of hours of humorous sitcoms on television, like "Friends" about people having relationships and humorous conversations about random things. I even tried memorising the dialogue'.

- 'Reading fiction has helped me to understand how people think and feel'.

- 'I've learned how to do attentive listening and make appropriate comments such as "Oh dear", or "How sad for you" or "Mmm" or just nodding'.

*Using different mediums to express emotions:* you don't always have to speak your emotions. Many people find it easier to explain how they feel by using text messages or email.

- 'I find typing a message online much easier than talking to somebody face-to-face'.

- 'I find that I can identify my feelings by playing certain pieces of music – I'm not very good at finding the words'.

- 'I dance to express my emotions – I find it a great release'.

- 'I have become better at verbalising my emotions but sometimes my facial expression doesn't match up'.

- 'I can't find words for my emotions but I can draw a picture. My feelings are like a jagged graph or the teeth of a saw'.

## Understanding and coping with 'meltdowns'

Not all autistic people have meltdowns, but many do. A meltdown by definition is an extreme, involuntary, emotional and behavioural response to a stressful situation – more than a behavioural outburst – that is usually caused by sensory, cognitive or social triggers. There are usually few warning signs. One moment the individual could be content and the next completely out of control. Although the diagnosed person themselves might not notice warning signs, an outsider might notice subtle signs such as more pressured speech, being slightly less coherent or an increase in repetitive behaviours. The reactions are invariably 'fight', 'flight' or 'freeze' and might be an explosion of frustration or anger, running away for self-preservation, tears or self-injurious behaviour – such as biting themselves on their forearm or banging their head, or a retreat into themselves such as sitting in the corner humming or carrying out some other repetitive behaviour. Sometimes it might be a small trivial event which is the last straw to tip the balance. The explosiveness of a meltdown seems to be because adrenaline, a stress hormone, is released too quickly. A large emotional reaction or meltdown, where feelings are vented briefly, helps clear the system – it is a failsafe, a release of all that pent-up adrenaline. The autistic person feels physically better afterwards and recovers quickly; however, they might feel intense feelings of remorse, embarrassment or shame. Others involved might continue to feel devastated, harbouring hurt feelings.

Rita reported that she had a meltdown at a music festival:

> I had been to a previous music festival and it had gone just about OK. I had planned meticulously and thought that I'd taken every precaution, making lists and back up plans but it all went wrong. I think it was a combination of a lack of sleep, too many people, too many

strangers who were friends of friends and it was just too social, too chaotic, out of control. I just flipped and was shaking, trembling, crying; I couldn't make sense and literally collapsed. People were trying to be helpful, getting me to walk. I just needed to be in a quiet dark comfortable place. I left the festival and felt better and just wanted to sleep.

*Recognise the potential triggers to a meltdown:*

- Novel situations or sudden unexpected changes or unplanned events.

- Sensory overload: loud noise, chaos, bright fluorescent lights, crowds, strong smells and people's touch (particularly when unexpected).

- Background stresses, e.g. transitions from school to work, moving to a new house or changing jobs.

- Being time pressured, pushed or hurried.

- Conversations, including sub-conversations or multiple people talking.

- Communication where people are vague, non-specific or imprecise, saying things such as, 'How do you feel?', or 'Just a minute', or offering vague instructions or open-ended questions.

- Social contact where there is no time limit or escape.

*When trying to help someone in meltdown, avoid the following as it might inflame the situation:*

- Don't raise your voice.

- Don't ask the person 'What's wrong?' – the person probably won't know, or they may not be able to articulate this.

- Don't ask questions or offer choices.

- Don't use sarcasm.

- Don't use physical restraint or touch the person without permission.

- Don't move in too close without prior approval.

*Instead:*

- Use a quiet but assertive voice and focus on distraction or a more constructive way of releasing the energy.

- Encourage the person to have some time out or solitude to calm down.

- Encourage engagement with some physical activity to burn it off or engage in their own strategy such as self-stimming.

- Reassure the person that these intense feeling will go.

- Don't try and 'fix the problem' by offering instruction.

- It may help the person just to be a presence and say nothing or offer a short reassuring phrase, such as, 'It's going to be OK'.

*Tips for coping with meltdowns (for client):*

- Try to identify the stressors and triggers for meltdowns. Sensory, cognitive or social? Can any of them be prevented or reduced?

- Devise your own 'stress thermometer' and regularly rate your level of stress from 0 to 100.

- Try to become aware of overload and regulate and plan your life so that you are not overwhelmed. Think ahead, have a plan and prepare.

- Have a stress level repair kit, this might be listening to your favourite music on headphones or inhaling a soothing smell or playing a game on your phone or having a favourite texture or object to touch.

- Follow a proper diet, get enough sleep and commune with nature.

- Engage in physical movement or exercise to vent and release/burn off adrenaline.

- Try to correct the underlying cause of the meltdown by reducing the stimulation levels – remove yourself from the underlying cause of the problem.

- Breathe deeply and count to 10, which is simple but sometimes effective.

- Have an escape strategy – go somewhere to be alone or do something to de-stress.

- Talk to somebody, emotionally unburden yourself and allow the listener to piece it all together.

- Seek advice – it helps to share a problem.

## The social world and socialising – 'I fill up quickly'

For many autistic people, socialising does not come naturally. It is often an effort and can be tiring. Asperger (1944, p58) said,

> Normal children acquire the necessary social habits without being consciously aware of them, they learn instinctively. It is these instinctive social relations that are disturbed in autistic children. Social adaptation has to proceed via the intellect.

There is a clash of culture between the autistic and non-autistic worlds over socialising. Some autistic people might perceive people in the non-autistic world as social zealots, prioritising socialising above anything else and expecting everybody to find socialising easy, natural and rewarding.

There is a paradox in that socialising and friendship can be one of the biggest insulators against stress, low mood and low self-esteem. It can also protect from real or perceived threats and help with problem solving. But at the same time, friendships can be one of the biggest causes of stress and depression. A compromise is needed between the two cultures.

## Capacity for socialising – 'I fill up quickly'

We all have different capacities for socialising; some people are naturally intuitively comfortable in a social situation, whereas for others it requires effort and energy. Generally speaking, people on the spectrum tend to feel more comfortable if social interactions are brief, purposeful and have a fixed ending as they need to go away and recharge their batteries. Willey (1999, p43) commented about her level or desire for socialisation, 'To me friends were people I enjoyed a few minutes or a few hours with... I fill up quickly'.

James, a client, commented,

> I actually like some social situations as long as they are time limited and preferably structured. So, meeting for a purpose like to play a game is better than just meeting to "chill out" or be at a party. But after a while I'm used up, spent, I've said what I want to say and need a break, some restoration time, time on my own. I can do social-ising but two hours is my maximum. It helps to know when it's going to be over.

Solitude is a natural state for many autistic people and is also the most effective emotional restorative, a way of calming down. It is understandable why many young autistic men retreat to the sanctuary and refuge of their bedroom, with online computer games.

Socialising involves numerous skills, particularly the art of 'small talk'. Imagine the situation – a group of people are waiting to start a course, or milling around at a party. What are the skills involved in starting a conversation? First, reading the other person's face and body language to see whether they are friendly, approachable and want to engage in conversation: what mood are they in, what is their intention? Starting a conversation involves thinking of something to say, stringing a few sentences together – an opener – which could be a question or at least something appropriate. Their words need to be matched with a friendly demeanour, appropriate facial expressions, gestures and tone of voice. Then there is responding to the other person's talk, keeping the conversation going, straying into and sharing mutual areas of interest. This involves recognising that the other person might not want to talk about a particular special interest and picking up the cues that they might be bored. Then there is the business of subtly and lightly disengaging and moving off and talking to somebody else.

The subtle art of socialising involves that key skill of being able to do two things at the same time. Simultaneously being able to listen, respond non-verbally with eye contact, nod and grunt if required, formulate your own feelings and responses and then deliver that response appropriately, in 'synch' with the other person. It is important for people with autism to know the rules and reasons behind social behaviour – to understand the logic. I remember one autistic lady called Theresa who was in the Territorial Army and used to go away at weekends, I assumed this would involve a lot of stressful socialising. She enlightened me by saying, 'Socialising in the army officers' mess is much easier than anywhere I've ever come across, as there are specific rules about who you speak to and how you speak'.

## Friendship – 'A Raven in a World of Crows'

Friendships and relationships are complicated, emotional and unpredictable, which is very challenging for autistic people who often report having few friendships. They may struggle to maintain relationships and enjoy less satisfying social lives than neurotypicals.

Autistic people can usually function reasonably well in a one-to-one social situation, often having one good friend, but when things get more complicated and there are three or four people, difficulties become more apparent – 'two's company, three's a crowd'. I recently attended an autism conference where one young autistic speaker called Ally, gave a brilliant talk entitled, 'A Raven in a World of Crows'. This metaphor illustrates the fact that you often see a flock of crows circling around in the sky, always in groups, (like her schoolgirl colleagues), whereas ravens are inevitably seen together in pairs – something I never realised! Difficulties in groups may arise if the person has slower information processing skills and is unable to process all the necessary social cues fast enough to stay synchronised with the conversation of the group. They might not be able to switch attention rapidly from one speaker to the next and might get left behind. One person reported that in a group situation, she would often find herself not being able to keep up and having to refer back saying, 'Going back to what you were just saying, I think ...'

Autistic people have certain qualities that make them good friends and partners. They can be undeniably loyal, trustworthy, dependable, honest and truthful, straightforward, confident about their opinions, relatively independent, happy to amuse themselves, usually calm, rational, dependable in a crisis and happy to share practical knowledge. They can be compassionate towards others as are likely to have been the victim of teasing and bullying themselves. They don't need to gossip or pry into the affairs of others and are often committed to the best interest of others.

## School, bullying and finding a mentor

School is often a stressful and mentally exhausting environment where autistic children have to work harder than other children because they not only have to cope with academic demands, but social demands as well. They are people who need a break, a period of solitude to recharge their batteries, and are often found in a quiet room, the library or, for example, the chess club.

Research suggests that children on the autism spectrum are bullied 4 times more than neurotypical children and that 90% of mothers of autistic children reported that their child had been bullied. Stories of being the last person picked for sports teams or wandering around the playground on their own are common. They don't have a protective network, are socially naive and eager to be part of a group and have poor social antennae for identifying the predators. One man said,

> I was bullied at school, but the main problem was that I couldn't see it coming. People would ask me questions, some to wind me up maliciously, but others might genuinely want to know. I couldn't discern which were genuine and which were a wind-up – I couldn't pick the good guys from the bad guys.

Teenage autistic girls are particularly vulnerable to sexual exploitation due to their naiveté, or lack of social antennae, where they don't recognise that the intentions of others might be sexual or malevolent. It helps to have a mentor. Willey (1999, p40) touchingly describes a boy called Craig who throughout her school career offered mentorship and protection: 'Craig jumped in to rescue me even before I knew I needed to be rescued'. Willey suggests that everybody with autism in the school situation would benefit from a mentor/protector figure like Craig.

*Ways of coping with the social world (clients' comments):*

- 'My mother took me along to a drama group at the age of twelve, which was the best decision we ever made as I learned so much about social skills and how to act in social situations. I learned about body language, facial expression, tone of voice, and how to respond in a variety of complex social situations'.

- 'I have learnt a lot about social skills from watching soap operas on television'.

- 'I think it's easier to join a special interest group, or a group where there is a common subject to talk about, like cycling or photography – conversation is easier'.

- 'Working with animals is a good way to meet like-minded people. I think a fair few autistic people are specially tuned into animals – it's a skill we have. I'm rubbish at communicating with people, but good with animals'.

- 'I do Taekwondo because it increases skills in self-protection, acts as a deterrent against bullying and also helps teach skills about remaining calm. It is also a rather solitary sport, which requires a great deal of structured repetition and practice, often ideal for somebody with autistic traits'.

- 'I use the internet to link up with people who might have a similar special interest'.

- 'I would suggest approaching people who have room for and value an extra friend, not somebody who is already too busy and popular'.

- 'I time limit my socialising. I went to a leaving "do", but said, "I'm only staying for an hour" and immediately felt better'.

- 'I try to develop the right degree of intensity by building friendships gradually. I used to be too intense and sometimes scared the other person off. Similarly, I try not to be too shy; otherwise the other person might think I'm not interested'.

## Marriage and romantic partnerships

In many ways, autistic people have the qualities to build a successful partnership. They are likely to have a way of thinking that focusses on being logical, pragmatic and straightforward rather than emotional. If there is a problem, the autistic approach is more likely to be practical, 'Let's try to find a way to fix it and make each other happy', rather than having moodiness, hidden subterranean feelings, drama, sulking, volatility and lingering resentments. They are also likely to be honest, loyal and happy to be alone, quite capable of occupying their own time with their special interest, rather than being 'clingy or dependent'. One autistic lady commented, 'My relationship is crucial to me: my partner is also my best friend. But I never miss him when we are apart – I usually forget about him completely when I'm busy at work'.

Hendrickx (2015, p178) in talking about her partner, who is also autistic (but neither knew at the time they met), describes their relationship as being like two peas in a pod:

> We can happily spend 24 hours a day together for extended periods… we place few emotional demands on each other and any that are placed are explicitly defined, avoiding uncertainty, anxiety or potential for failure… most importantly we accept each other without judgement regardless of how odd or unfathomable our behaviour is. As a woman with autism this has been a once-in-a-lifetime experience, a respite from the performance I put on for the rest of the world, a place to truly call "home".

However, there are obvious problems that make a romantic relationship difficult as the autistic partner might prefer more solitude and time alone rather than in intimacy. They may have special interests that give them satisfaction, rather than the quality of the interpersonal relationship itself, may prefer structure rather than spontaneity and may not pick up on the emotional needs of their partner. The most common complaint of a non-autistic partner married to a person with autism is that they feel lonely and miss out on regular affectionate affirmations, gestures or loving words. One distressed autistic lady married to a non-autistic man recently came to our clinic with the following warning:

> My husband said he wants a divorce after 17 years of marriage. I really don't want that and need to find a way of saving my marriage. He says he feels "at the bottom of the pile" because I put my interests first and don't show enough affection. I have let my interest in Alternative Reality games and *Pokemon Go* take over. He hates it. I get up at six o'clock in the morning and play for a few hours before work then again after work, I'm there until about 11.0 o'clock. He wanted children but I never did – I never found the idea interesting and he had concerns about how good I'd be as a Mum. I'm really trying to reduce my game playing to save our marriage.

Relationships between somebody on the spectrum and a neurotypical person are often complex. There might be an attraction of opposites – both give something different which makes a whole – in simplistic terms, one does most of the thinking and the other more of the feeling. The neurotypical partner might also have a role as the 'executive secretary', helping with organisational problems and planning, and also acting as the social secretary. It is noticeable that many autistic people have sympathetic, understanding, partners – often people who work in the caring professions, such as nurses, counsellors or social workers – who offer a degree of emotional support, mentoring and guidance in the social world.

Most autistic people have a desire and need for an intimate relationship (it is only a small percentage that would not fall into that category). They have strong feelings and a great capacity to love, but the lack of social skills to build a relationship and the difficulty reading other people's emotions often creates challenges.

The Asperger Couple's Workbook, by Aston (2009), gives practical advice and useful strategies to help couples in a relationship where one partner is autistic. She makes the point that communication is a major problem as both partners are on a different wavelength and speak a different language. One is logical and linear, taking one subject at a time, and the other is likely to be more emotional and unpredictable. Some useful tips include the following:

• No distractions: if having an important conversation, make sure the TV and radio are off, there are no other people present, you are not eating or driving and you have time.

- The colour communication system: this is a visual form of communicating rather than using words because words can be hurtful, or difficult, particularly in the heat of an argument. The couple can use actual coloured cards, like a set of traffic lights or the referee's card used in football. A red card stands for danger, meaning, 'We need to stop; pause this debate as I'm frightened it will get out of control'. A yellow card stands for uncertainty, meaning, 'I don't fully understand what you mean; please can we go back and you tell me in a way I can understand'. A green card means, 'I'm OK with what you have told me. I understand'.

- The anger thermometer: visualise a thermometer with a 10-point scale and when anger or frustration increases, the red liquid rises up the scale towards 10. If a couple are having a disagreement and one partner is feeling frustrated, they could simply interject, 'My thermometer is at 8', which informs the other that it's time to pause and diffuse the tension.

- Rules for socialising: it is sometimes helpful if the couple have a prearranged agreement or series of coded signs for communication when socialising. So, for example, a pinch or a movement of finger to lip might mean, 'Stop saying what you are saying immediately'. A wink might mean, 'You are doing very well'. If the autistic person is feeling overloaded by the situation, they could say, 'I think I have a migraine coming on', as an excuse to leave.

## The effect of diagnosis on marriage and romantic partnerships

A diagnosis not only affects the person themselves but also the relationship they might be in. In romantic partnerships or marriages, where one member is autistic and the other is neurotypical, reactions can vary. The general consensus seems to be that a diagnosis represents a positive change, aiding understanding, improving coping and strengthening the relationship. However, on rarer occasions, the diagnosis might not make the relationship stronger. There follows three different stories from neurotypical partners, who explain their reaction when their partner received a diagnosis of autism.

Michael, married to Gill who obtained a late-in-life autism diagnosis, tells his story:

> Before getting the diagnosis, we'd been married for five years and used to have lots of arguments. The diagnosis has helped me understand Gill more and we've gradually worked it out. When we used to get into a conversation about emotions, Gill would stop talking, start to pace up and down, cry and wring her hands. I would get

angry with her and say something cruel like, "Grow up, you're an adult" and sometimes walk out slamming the door. Now I know she just can't process emotions the way other people do. I say to myself, "She can't help it", and stay calm. I then try to explain myself in a rational manner because that makes sense to Gill. Sometimes she needs to type an answer and we will sit on the sofa texting each other. I also now know Gill needs a set routine in the morning. Everything has to be done the same way. I don't speak to her for the first 20 minutes; then I'll bring her a cup of coffee just as she likes it. Now that I know how her mind works, I can appreciate it – she communicates rationally in logic and fact. I love her for the way she is, different from everybody else. She's unique, brilliant and honest and I believe we challenge each other and are growing into better people.

A different story comes from Vanessa, a non-autistic lady married to Alan, who obtained a diagnosis 3 years ago:

I must say that getting the diagnosis for Alan was a turning point for me and our 15-year marriage, which has always been difficult. For Alan it was brilliant, a validation of the way he was, but I began to see him as a different person. I began to see more and more how he was preoccupied with his work and his hobbies and I felt neglected and unloved. When pushed, he would show some affection, but I knew he was only going through the motions. I don't think he really felt it. I realised that he would never change. His brain was wired up logically and I know he loved me in his rational way and was totally loyal, but I'm more emotional and our worlds were drifting apart. The more I became depressed, the more he failed to connect with me. What made it worse was that I could see our son, who also has autism, slowly changing and becoming more empathic with the help he was getting at school, but Alan wasn't. I started chatting to a male friend at work who was going through a divorce and I realised that a man could be emotional and sensitive. This has created problems because I feel torn.

A further story from stand-up comedian Amy Schumer, from her live show, talking about her husband getting an autism diagnosis:

All the characteristics that make it clear he is on the spectrum are all the reasons I fell madly in love with him. He says whatever is on his mind. He keeps it so real. He doesn't care about social norms, or what you expect him to say or do…he can't live a lie. Is that the dream man?…The tools that we have been given have made his life so much better and our marriage so much manageable. …so I just want to encourage people not to be afraid of stigma.

## Sexuality

Sexuality for people on the spectrum is often complex for a variety of reasons, including sensory sensitivities, communication and emotional issues. One study (Bejerot and Erikson, 2014) compared autistic people with matched controls, finding that for autistic males and females there was generally a lower level of libido than for controls. There were also higher rates of 'tomboyism', 'bisexuality' and 'asexuality' in the female autism group; lower gender identification... less 'girly girly' behaviour. For men, particularly young men, the issue might be trying to find a sexual partner, where poor social skills, difficulty communicating, flirting, 'reading signals' and maintaining a relationship can be a problem, resulting in real frustration.

A further study (Pecora et al 2019) interviewed 135 autistic women, 161 neurotypical women and 96 autistic men about their sexual experiences. They confirmed the theory that autistic women tend to be less interested in sex than autistic men. Yet they also found that autistic women have had more sexual experiences than autistic men do. However, many of them report regretting these experiences, identifying them as being abusive or not having wanted them in the first place. According to that study, autistic women are more likely to have been sexually abused or victimised than neurotypical women, perhaps because they are often more vulnerable, they don't pick up on the intentions of predatory individuals and fail to recognise or report abuse. However, it might be that those negative or unwanted experiences are a factor that contributes to a reduced interest.

Gillan Drew, author of the book, 'An Adult with an Autism Diagnosis' (2017, p138–140) makes the following observation about the role of imagination and sensory sensitivities and the art of sex:

> In my (limited) experience, people on the autism spectrum can be unimaginative when it comes to sex. As with most social acts, sex requires effective communication and the ability to understand the needs of the other person, and struggling in these areas, people with autism can therefore interpret sex in a goal orientated, functional manner, as a mechanism for pleasure rather than a complex emotional bonding experience between two people. Focusing on the genitals and the act of penetration until climax... the autistic partner can lack an appreciation of the surrounding features of sex, such as emotional closeness, intimacy, foreplay, experimentation, the art of romance, cuddling, kissing, paying attention to other parts of the body and an intuitive meeting of the partner's desires. This is not to say we are bad or selfish lovers, and we can learn about sex intellectually... but it is not something that comes naturally to us... Some people with autism can be extremely sensitive to touch or stimulation and struggle to contain their feelings when being cuddled or stroked and to those people sex is an intolerable thought. The sight, sounds, smell, taste and touch of sex can be overwhelming, bewildering and unpleasant.

For autistic women, married to non-autistic men, there might be potential problems. One married lady with autism commented, 'I'm not really interested in sex and don't really want it. But my logical brain says I should be doing it to keep my husband happy'. Emma, a recently diagnosed 30-year-old, commented, 'I'm asexual and aromantic. I don't feel sexual or romantic feelings. In fact, I'm repulsed'. Temple Grandin said, 'My sense of self and happiness is tied up with what I do, my career, and I don't need or want an intimate sexual relationship'. Tony Attwood suggested, in a recent presentation, an interesting thought – in Europe, a 1000 years ago, the monasteries where men found pleasure in routine, solitary activities and celibacy were probably full of people with autism!

Sexual relations can have a dual function – first, a purely physical functional basis or a desire to satisfy a sexual desire or need; second, a desire for emotional intimacy, to enhance the quality of a relationship. There is some evidence that sexual relations in autism can be more functional and less imbided with emotional intimacy. One recently diagnosed young lady commented,

> I probably see the emotional and physical side of sexual interaction as separate from each other, more like a man would. To me, sex is a basic animal instinct that has to be satisfied like hunger or sleep and often I don't see the need for a partner. However, I do like men and I've probably been a bit promiscuous in terms of boyfriends, but I feel that with sex it is something I have to offer, it is something that I can bring to the table... make a contribution in a friendship or relationship. In some ways it's actually easier than having a lengthy conversation.

# CHAPTER 7

# Mental health and related issues

## Neurodevelopmental and psychiatric overlapping diagnosis (co-morbidities)

Autism overlaps with a number of other neurodevelopmental and psychiatric conditions. Neurodevelopmental conditions, largely conditions that people are born with, due to the 'wiring of the brain', include attention deficit hyperactivity disorder (ADHD), dyslexia, dyspraxia, dyscalculia, Tourette's syndrome, learning difficulties and epilepsy. On top of these shared conditions, both children and adults with autism are more vulnerable to secondary mental health conditions, such as anxiety, depression, low self-esteem, obsessive–compulsive disorder (OCD), eating disorders, psychosis, bipolar disorder, addictions trauma/post-traumatic stress disorder and personality disorders. Then there is gender dysphoria (GD), which is more common in autistic people, which for convenience I have put in this chapter (See Figure 7.1). It is easy to imagine how the social, emotional, behavioural and sensory struggles of living with autism, whether diagnosed or not, can lead to secondary mental health problems. Almost eight in ten autistic adults experience a mental health problem (Tromsans et al, 2018). Up to 10% of adults in psychiatric inpatient settings are autistic even though only 1% of the general population is on the spectrum (Lever and Geurts, 2016). Ongoing research suggests that up to 10% of people who die by suicide may be autistic and autistic women are markedly more likely to die by suicide than men (Hirvikoski et al, 2016). There is also the problem of individuals being misdiagnosed with other psychiatric conditions such as schizophrenia or borderline personality disorder, when the underlying problem is autism.

The risk factors that can influence the likelihood of a person with autism having mental health problems include the following:

1 Inherent difficulties in recognising, expressing and regulating emotions.

2 Limited friendship and social networks; less likely to have someone to

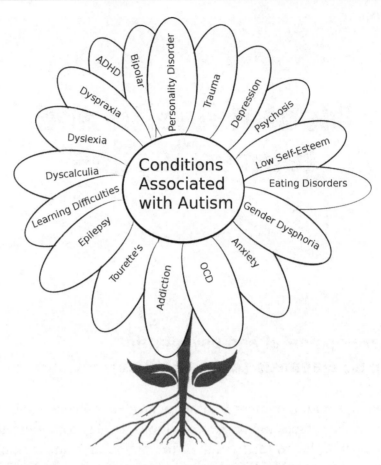

*Figure 7.1* Neurodevelopmental and secondary psychiatric conditions associated with autism (co-morbidities)

confide in or receive advice and social support.

3 Lack of opportunities to access work or meaningful reinforcing activities.

4 Difficulty coping with certain environments because of sensory or social difficulties (e.g. school, open plan offices etc.).

5 Increased vulnerability to bullying, abuse and trauma in both childhood and adulthood.

6 Thinking style can be concrete – all or nothing – which correlates with depression.

7 Not receiving a diagnosis in childhood, so the person has no explanation for their struggles, in their developmental years.

## Primary neurodevelopmental co-morbidities

### ADHD

The most common co-morbidity with autism is ADHD, sometimes presenting in a less active form as attention deficit disorder (ADD), without the hyperactivity. The general condition of ADHD affects between 3 and 5% of the general population. It is characterised by: (1) hyperactivity, being fidgety, 'on the go', restless and finding it difficult to relax; (2) impulsivity: acting before thinking; and (3) difficulty concentrating, being unable to filter out background information, or split and divide attention. People with ADHD get bored very easily, need a high level of stimulation and can be forgetful and disorganised, often talking excessively. Approximately 10–14% of people with autism would meet the criteria for ADHD or ADD. People with subclinical levels of both autism and ADHD may miss out on a full diagnosis of either condition but can still be significantly disadvantaged due to the combination of symptoms.

Two clients' comments are revealing as follows:

- 'It's like there are two voices in my head or two horses pulling in different directions; one wants me to be obsessive and develop special interests and really focus on something, but the other is restless and pulls me away – I just don't have the patience to develop an all-encompassing autistic type special interest'.

- 'Having both ASD and ADHD is a double whammy for me. The ADHD means that I can't keep my mouth shut, can't stop talking and the ASD means that what comes out of my mouth is often too honest, inappropriate, blunt and rude'.

## Dyspraxia

This is a condition characterised by difficulties in two main areas – first, problems with gross and/or fine motor skills, eye–hand coordination and clumsiness; as a child, there are often marked delays in learning to walk, poor ball skills, poor coordination with tasks such as riding a bicycle, tying a knot in a tie or a bow in shoelaces and often poor handwriting, and second, difficulties with executive functioning, such as organising and planning, memory, multitasking and sequential activities. Approximately 90% of people with dyspraxia have another neurodevelopmental disorder such as autism or ADHD.

## Tourette's syndrome

Prevalence rates are estimated as being between 0.15 and 1.8% of the general population. The condition is characterised by a tic – an involuntary, rapid, recurrent, non-rhythmic, motor or vocal action which is sudden and purposeless. About 10% of autistic people have vocal or motor tics. Simple tics can include eye blinking or rolling, facial grimacing, shoulder shrugging, tongue protrusions, knuckle cracking, throat clearing, grunting and making different meaningless sounds. More complex tics might include gyrating, touching objects, swearing or repeating certain words or phrases. Between 20 and 60% of autistic people have tics or involuntary, repetitive contractions of groups of muscles (including the vocal cords). In those with autism, tics tend to wax and wane with degrees of stress and depression.

## Dyslexia/hyperlexia

Dyslexia is defined as having difficulty with literacy or words which might include reading, spelling and writing. People with dyslexia often have a reduced working memory (the ability to retain information over a very short period of time, often a matter of seconds). The opposite of dyslexia is hyperlexia meaning a superability or precocious ability to read and decode words often without understanding their meaning. The child might remember and read the word but not understand its meaning. Both dyslexia and hyperlexia are common in autism. One study suggested 5–10% of autistic children to be hyperlexic.

## Dyscalculia

While the majority of people with autism are proficient with numbers and figures, some are very poor and simply can't do arithmetic, taking years to learn to add, subtract, divide and multiply or tell the time. Some autistic people really struggle with the concept of time and with placing events chronologically, while others are exceptionally good in this area.

## Epilepsy

One in four children with 'classic autism' and a learning disability have a seizure disorder. For adults, the prevalence rate is thought to be about 12%. Seizures can range from full-scale convulsions to brief staring spells. However, little is known about the prevalence rates in the 'milder' condition of Asperger's.

## Learning disability (LD)

A high proportion of people with very severe autism have a learning disability (LD); research suggests this is as high as 50%. However, autistic people may get misdiagnosed as having an LD when actually they just have an unusual cognitive profile, being very strong in certain skills and very weak in others (See Figure 7.2).

## Secondary psychiatric difficulties

## Anxiety

Experiencing anxiety is by far the most common and highest rated problem for autistic people. There are at least four major root causes: (1) difficulty socialising with the continuous possibility of making mistakes and feeling humiliated; (2) intolerance of uncertainty and the stress of coping with unpredictability, unknown, unexpected events and changes to routine; (3) the stress of sensory experiences and sensory overload such as overwhelming noise, light, smell and (4) special fears or phobias such as of telephones, heights, the dark or large dogs.

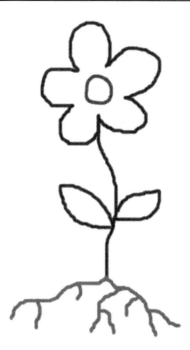

*Figure 7.2* 'Misdiagnosis is often about looking at the petals, rather than the roots'. The roots or primary diagnosis can often be autism

Experiencing anxiety is a vicious circle as the more anxious a person feels, the more they tighten up and become rigid, leading to socialising becoming more difficult and more impinging sensory issues. Then the person avoids, escapes or doesn't cope, which creates more anxiety next time around, resulting in a negative feedback loop, an escalation or a vicious circle. Typical ways of coping with anxiety might include (1) escape, avoidance, refusal, social phobia and solitude; (2) engaging in routine, rituals and special interests in an attempt to make the world more controllable and predictable; (3) taking prescription medication, alcohol and drugs; (4) freezing – selective mutism. Most of these strategies produce short-term benefits in relief from anxiety, but some, if used to excess, have the potential to store up added long-term difficulties.

The condition of 'social anxiety' or 'social phobia' in non-autistic people is in some ways similar but in some ways different from that experienced by autistic people. The non-autistic person with social anxiety often has only a mild social skill difficulty but has an excessive amount of avoidance, catastrophising and anxiety, whereas the person with autism often has a much bigger social skill difficulty.

*Tips for coping with anxiety:*

- Try to work out what triggers and causes your anxiety. Write a list so you will be able to anticipate and plan for situations.

- Have a place to go, a sanctuary or retreat, where there is minimum stimulation and you can be alone and de-stress.

- Take care of yourself with a good diet, plenty of sleep and exercise that raises your heartbeat.

- Learn coping strategies such as relaxation techniques, mindfulness or breathing exercises. Try to fill your mind with a soothing picture.

- Use distractions – immerse yourself in your special interest.

- Learn to forgive yourself for your mistakes – no one is perfect – we are all struggling. Focus on your strong points.

## Depression

Depression is common because, not only do autistic people have difficulty getting social needs met, but also they have reduced social support and work opportunities and often have experienced bullying and abuse. Andrews (2006) suggests that anxiety and depression in people with autism are responses to two main problems in society: societal pressure to conform and societal hostility towards those who are different. Additionally, autistic people often have perfectionistic tendencies and sometimes have difficulty resonating with and infusing happiness from others; also having a brain that is prone to rumination and repetition, particularly around negative thoughts. In autism, depression is sometimes experienced in an unconventional way because the person has difficulty understanding and expressing emotions and may not hang on to lingering unhappy emotions from the past. Rather than a prolonged period of sustained gloom the person might have a briefer 'depression attack', rather like a panic attack, which can come quickly, be intense and overwhelming and then go quickly. This leaves the person vulnerable to self-harm, suicidal thoughts and even suicide. Cassidy et al (2014) indicated that autistic people are more prone to suicidal ideation (ideas in the mind/brain) than the general population and have more risk factors for depression. Wylie (2015, p111) commented, 'Suicidal thinking is a non-emotional, logical, analysis of the situation: suicide is one of the potential options'. Black and white thinking with no grey areas in the middle can mean that moods switch from one extreme to the other very quickly.

Some people on the spectrum seem to have generally low capacity for pleasure and reward in life; the dopamine pathways in areas of the brain are simply not very active. There is a condition called 'anhedonia', which means, 'the inability to experience pleasure from activity usually found enjoyable, such as eating, exercise, social interaction and sexual experiences'. Some people say they experience anhedonia, although others say they get a great deal of pleasure from their special interests and a few more say they experience pleasure but not from social situations. Thomas's story illustrates this point:

> I don't have needs or an appetite; everything is a means to an end. I'll be glad when it's all over. My wife said let's go on holiday and I think, "Why, what's the point". I do things to make my wife happy. I try to be a good provider and husband – and I suppose that is a sort

of vicarious pleasure, but I don't need any of it. I never look forward to anything whether it be a new car, birthday, holiday or Christmas ... it's just another day. I have no need for friends. Social interaction is like a game which I will play for a while and then come home and play with my cars. I don't get any pleasure out of physical contact. Linda says, "Let's have a cuddle on the settee", and I think, what for?

*Tips for coping with depression:*

- Get to know yourself. Learning about autism can make sense of years of frustration and baffling failure.

- Stop blaming yourself. One man said, 'The more I understand about autism the more I realise it's not my fault ... my brain is just wired up differently'.

- Keep busy and have routines and interests. Immersing yourself in a special interest or taking on a caring role for others, or having a pet, shifts your attention away from negative thoughts.

- Understand and express yourself through music, art or creative channels.

- Ensure you allot time for exercise, good diet, communing with nature and taking an active interest in the environment.

- Develop a spiritual interest – an awareness of a higher purpose putting self into context.

- Consider seeking professional help, perhaps from a psychological therapist with knowledge of autism.

## Low self-esteem

Autistic people often have problems with low self-esteem because they feel different growing up: experiencing bullying, criticism from peers, lack of friends and self-criticism from making mistakes. Paul said, 'I've always felt different, like I'm not good enough. I try to keep below the radar, be unnoticed'. Shame or the fear that one is being negatively judged in the eyes of others is an accompanying partner to low self-esteem.

*Tips for coping with poor self-esteem:*

- Accept that difference is not defective. Accepting yourself just as you are makes it more likely that others will accept you.

- Write two lists. In the first, think of aspects about yourself that you are proud of or that people have complimented you on, for example, your honesty and loyalty. Then, in the second list, identify your abilities or things that you are good at, for example, memory or an eye for detail. It may help to ask family and friends to help you complete the list.

- Remind yourself that you are doing your best and that you are not a 'bad person'.

- Find like-minded people who have similar interests or characteristics like you. For example, there may be a group of people who also go to 'Dr Who' or 'Star Trek' conventions and play the same computer games.

- Spend time with nature, animals or pets. Some autistic people often have special abilities to commune with animals, which can be a great boost to self-esteem.

- Identify the value of being different. Read about autistic achievers in the science and arts.

## Schizophrenia or psychosis

Research suggests that autistic people have 3–4 times greater risk of developing signs of schizophrenia than non-autistic people (Zheng et al, 2018). The relationship between autism and schizophrenia has been tortuous and right up until the late 1970s, autism was known as 'childhood schizophrenia' and this shared history still causes confusion and misdiagnosis. Autistic people do appear to be particularly prone to brief psychotic episodes classically induced by severe stress. Young autistic adults in particular can develop genuine signs of schizophrenia, such as hearing voices, delusions or paranoia, but often such episodes tend to be transient and linked to stressful events. It is important, if it is a transient state, for this to be recognised and the patient not carry an unnecessary diagnosis of schizophrenia for years.

There can also be confusion and misdiagnosis as some of the more negative indicators of autism can resemble symptoms of schizophrenia, such as poor social communication skills, social withdrawal, unusual disorganised thinking, self-neglect, lack of personal hygiene, poverty of affect and bizarre behaviour. Furthermore, in both schizophrenia and autism, the person might vocalise their thoughts or talk about themselves in the third person or be suspicious of others. A further factor is that autistic people often have usual sensory experiences and, for example, might continue to see an image from TV after it has gone or continue to hear a voice, almost as an after image.

Differentiating between the negative symptoms of schizophrenia, or 'schizoid personality disorder', and autism can be challenging. One obvious differentiating factor is that for a diagnosis of schizophrenia, there has to be a progressive loss of social contact, social functioning, and general deterioration in functioning in areas such as work and self-care, whereas, in those with autism, the general level of functioning remains constant as there never has been extensive social contact. The key to a good assessment is to look at the person's early neurodevelopmental history and have a reliable informant, such as a

*Table 7.1* Similarities and differences between schizophrenia and autism

| Symptom | Schizophrenia | Autism |
| --- | --- | --- |
| Onset | Childhood usually normal – onset early adulthood. | Autistic symptoms – from very early age (before 10 years). |
| Hallucinations | Hearing voices, which the person is unable to control – often reluctant to discuss, wants them to go away. Often out of touch with reality. | Often escapes into imaginary world… imaginary friends. Can get after images or voices from TV, (eidetic imagery). Could be misinterpretation of an internal dialogue. Often happy to discuss experiences. Knows they are not real. Still in touch with reality. |
| Delusions/paranoia | Fixed irrational beliefs in one area of life – reluctant to discuss. Generally, rigid beliefs not associated with other areas of life. | High level of paranoia linked to 'black and white thinking' and 'jumping to conclusions' e.g. 'People are talking about me'. Rigid beliefs generalised to most areas of life rather than one area – but autistic people mostly happy to discuss. Delusions of grandiosity can be an extension of fantasy world. |
| Thought disorder | Disorganised thinking and speech, illogicality, and thought blocking. | Difficulty relating clear narrative – misses bits out, goes off on tangents and stuck on details. Sometimes giving too much detail. |
| Poverty of thought and speech | Either absence of thought or preoccupied with internal experience. | Can be slow processing speed, pedantic language, need to 'get it right'. |
| Poverty of affect (emotion or feeling) | Flat emotional range, but often a gradual deterioration in functioning over time. | Narrow range of emotions, slow to process emotions or lack of ability to articulate emotions. Poor non-verbal behaviours from early age. |
| Unusual special interests and skills | Not usually. | Areas of specialist skill and knowledge. Good eye for detail and memory. |
| Restricted repetitive behaviour, liking sameness | Not usually. | Usual. Lifelong liking of routine and rituals. Days planned. Does not like unexpected changes. |
| Sensory sensitivities | Infrequent apart from general sensory overload. | Frequent. Noise, light, touch, taste, texture, smell sensitivities or under sensitivities. |
| Motor clumsiness | Infrequent. | Frequent. |

parent, who can identify whether symptoms existed in childhood or if there has been deterioration. However, some autistic people do develop schizophrenia and the psychotic features are not 'transient' but are permanent. To help with differentiating between the two conditions Table 7.1 highlights some of the similarities and differences.

Three relevant client stories are as follows.

William, aged 36 years old, received a diagnosis of Asperger's syndrome in his late teens and has been case managed by a community mental health team (CMHT) for 10 years. He experiences 'transient episodes' of increased paranoia and bizarre behaviour. William had been bullied excessively at school, struggled to hold down a job or relationships, has had a number of admissions to psychiatric hospitals and been sectioned on occasion; he now takes a small dose of antipsychotic medication. He commented,

> I think my parents and the police overreact – I'm not psychotic. I'm just having a massive meltdown but I can get very paranoid. Ever since I was a child, I have hated loud noises or people banging things and can get quite paranoid about it. Recently we had a big family Christmas meal with about 12 people – I was already stressed before-hand. There were lots of little sub-conversations and my sister was banging things down on the table and I thought she was doing it deliberately. I stood up in the middle of the meal and started shouting and punched myself in the eye and ran off. They eventually found me and I was admitted to hospital again. I get paranoid about a number of things. For example, I often think my neighbour is deliberately making noise to get back at me or if people are sniffing or cough-ing in public, I think they are doing that to wind me up. This year I planned Christmas better so that I saw everybody individually or in small groups, with a gap between meetings, so I didn't have to sit down to one of those big family meals.

Sidney a 34-year-old man, who was referred from a CMHT for an autism assessment, is a good example of a misdiagnosis. He had been diagnosed with schizophrenia 12 years ago (aged 22), following one 'transient psychotic epi-sode' and had been taking antipsychotic drugs ever since. His mum queried the diagnosis, saying, 'It doesn't fit, he has worked consistently for 12 years doing a routine job in a printers, with no psychotic symptoms. I don't know why he's still on that medication'. Sidney was a quiet, shy man, of probable low average intelligence, who lived with his parents. On investigation, it appeared that the original incident, 12 years ago, had occurred when Sidney had become stressed by bullying work colleagues. He responded by sitting in the front window staring out into space for hours, fearfully saying 'People are after me', but he couldn't articulate his worries at the time. The treating psychiatrist diagnosed paranoia and schizophrenia and prescribed medica-tion. The compliant family had reluctantly accepted the diagnosis. After our assessment, Sidney was diagnosed with autism, the medication gradually reduced and then stopped to no ill effect.

A further example was a young man called Josh, who had been in a psychiatric ward for 8 weeks, with psychosis, which included grandiose delusions. The treating psychiatrist correctly thought he might have an underlying autism and referred him for an autism assessment. Josh was an insightful young man, who could articulately reflect back on his experiences and together we pieced together a possible link between his way of coping socially and the psychotic episode:

> I have always hated small talk … struggled to make friends and share with others. As a kid I used to retreat into my imagination and create my own fantasy world where I was always better than everybody

else. At university I put on this front of being really outgoing. I'd go to parties with my tribe and get absolutely plastered on drink and drugs. The psychotic episode occurred after a number of stresses and too many drugs. I thought I was 'the king of the world', that I'd been anointed and could do anything. The delusion was in some ways an extension of my childhood fantasies.

## Borderline personality disorder (BPD)/emotionally unregulated personality disorder (EUPD)/complex trauma (CT)

There is often misdiagnosis between autism and a cluster of conditions, variably named *borderline personality disorder (BPD)/emotionally unregulated personality disorder (EUPD) or complex trauma (CT)*. These conditions have common roots in attachment difficulties, exposure to interpersonal trauma, adverse experiences, invalidation, and psychological, sexual and physical abuse. A consequence of these negative experiences is that the person has difficulty regulating their emotions and maintaining mutually supportive relationships, developing unhelpful coping strategies. Misdiagnosis is common, particularly in women, where the 'female presentation' of autism is often misinterpreted.

Research by Lugnegard and colleagues, in 2011, identified 54 adults clinically diagnosed with autism but approximately half fulfilled the criteria for BPD. The confusion is understandable as both diagnoses have considerable overlaps and share similar characteristics:

- Severe mood swings or 'meltdowns' characterised by rage.

- Above-average number of suicidal thoughts and tendency to self-harm.

- Higher than average rate of bullying and childhood physical and/or sexual abuse.

- Tendency to 'black-and-white', 'all or nothing' thinking or 'splitting' where something is seen as completely good or completely bad, with the tendency to either idolise or vilify people.

- Stormy, difficult relationships, issues around intimacy, can hurt those closest to them – poor attachment styles.

- Feelings of emptiness and issues around self-identity.

- Alexithymia or difficulty identifying emotions and putting words to feelings.

However, there are very definite differences between the two conditions and, as with differentiating between autism and schizophrenia, the key is to carry out a detailed neurodevelopmental history.

Autism is from birth and is noticeable in early childhood, whereas the cluster of personality disorder diagnostic categories starts in late adolescence and early adulthood. The person with BPD generally knows how to make friends and has good social skills, but difficulty keeping relationships, whereas the person with autism has difficulty making friends and is more likely to have communication difficulties, use literal language and exhibit challenges interpreting non-verbal behaviour and humour. Furthermore, the person with BPD is also often highly sensitive to the moods and non-verbal behaviours of others, being highly attuned to picking up signs of rejection or criticism, whereas generally people with autism are less sensitive in this area. The person with autism is more likely to have hardwired sensory sensitivities (noise, light, touch, taste etc.) and motor coordination problems. A further generalisation borne out by research is that the person with autism often has a 'low openness to new practical and emotional experiences', meaning, they are not novelty or change seekers, but prefer sameness and routine, whereas the person with BPD often seeks change 'stimulation' and new experiences. Autistic people tend to be straightforward, honest, dutiful, with a frankness in expression, often adhering to the rules, with a tendency to think things through before acting, whereas the person with BPD is often more impulsive and less straightforward.

Ingrid had problems in relationships, was socially isolated, emotionally unstable, flying into frequent rages, self-harmed, and was rather prone to 'black-and-white' thinking. The local CMHT diagnosed her as having BPD. She was eventually referred for an assessment of autism, where one comment she made gave a decisive clue towards supporting an autism rather than BPD diagnosis. Ingrid said,

> When I was a child, my mother tried to help me, encouraging me to look at people rather than avoid eye contact. She also taught me how to cope better with social situations by understanding 'trick questions'. She said, people will say things like, "Do you like my jumper?" but they don't always want a truthful answer; these are trick questions. Since then I have tried to pick out trick questions and not take things so literally.

Eleanor had a long psychiatric history stretching back to childhood, including a history of extreme self-harm, teenage years in an adolescent unit, multiple forms of psychological therapy and a diagnosis of BPD. At the age of 25 years, she was referred to our autism assessment service. The following extracts from her interview are enlightening:

> I have a good relationship with both my parents... I'm told I started self-harming from the age of about two years – scratching my face and pulling my hair out. I think it was due to frustration. I hated noises like the hoover and I'm incredibly sensitive to heat. I started cutting at about twelve... I do it because of what I call 'brain static'.

I feel overwhelmed like a television or computer that has gone on the blink. Self-harming has become like an addiction, but I am always extremely well planned and organised and have researched anatomy so I know where all the arteries, nerves and veins are... Once I've done it, I feel calmer. It's like pressing the reset button on a computer; it clears all the apps and browsing history... I'm like my Borderline friends because of my 'black and white thinking', it's all or nothing, no half measures, but I'm different because I'm not impulsive or clingy and my triggers are different. My triggers are things like getting overwhelmed, heat, making a social mistake, unexpected events and shame... I also don't have romantic or sexual relationships, I'm not possessive or jealous and don't have issues around abandonment like them. I'm oblivious to all that. I like being on my own... I'm doing DBT (Dialectical Behavioural Therapy) with a number of people with Borderline and have found it very useful. I'm autistic first, but because of my self-harm, I'm told I've got both conditions.

There is a high rate of people with underlying autism being misdiagnosed with BPD. Receiving a correct diagnosis can often helpfully change the emphasis of psychological treatment. However, there are some people whose problems may be rooted in an underlying autism condition and then, because of significant trauma and attachment difficulties, may also have secondary features of complex trauma or borderline personality disorder. It is possible to have both diagnoses.

Table 7.2 illustrates the main similarities and differences between the two conditions, hopefully helping to make differential diagnosis easier.

## Obsessive–compulsive disorder (OCD)

There are many similarities between autism and OCD as both involve having rigid repetitive actions and routines and a narrow range of repetitive thoughts about a subject. Both groups have difficulty tolerating uncertainty and a tendency towards a concrete thinking style. Research suggests that between 8 and 20% of people with autism have a co-diagnosis of OCD. However, there are differences: the main difference being that in OCD, the intrusive or invasive thoughts are not welcome or wanted and bring enormous anxiety. This triggers a compulsive activity to neutralise the thought and reduce the anxiety – termed 'egodystonic'. In autism, the thoughts are quite pleasurable and the person does not have a desire to resist or stop having the thought – they are not coated with anxiety. Autistic people find comfort, flow and meaning in routine and ritual. The thoughts and repetitive activities might be part of a special interest and bring inherent pleasure and are not there to reduce anxiety. It is the function of, or reason behind, the repetitive compulsive patterns which are different in both conditions.

*Table 7.2* Similarities and differences between borderline personality disorder and autism

| Characteristic | BPD/EUPD/CT | Autism |
|---|---|---|
| Cause | Poor attachment, trauma, abuse, invalidating environments. | Hardwiring of brain. |
| Onset | Adolescence – early adulthood. | Very early childhood (<10 years). |
| Emotional sensitivity | Highly sensitive to others' emotional states (tone of voice, anger, emotional change etc.). Hyper-alert to potential emotional rejection, criticism or abandonment. | May not recognise emotions in others and poor at picking up emotional cues or non-verbal behaviours in others. When the person does pick up emotional cues, unsure how to respond. |
| Social | No difficulty in initiating conversation unless in emotional state. Knows how to make friends. Pattern of unstable, intense relationships. | Poor at initiating and managing reciprocal conversations. Lack of social understanding from an early age. Poor at making friends and small talk. Prefers one to one social situations. |
| Being alone/dependency | Often fear of being alone – dependent, clingy relationships. | Appreciates aloneness – not often emotionally clingy or dependent. |
| Emotional range | Intense emotional 'roller coaster'. Shares and talks about emotions freely. Emotionally rich vocabulary. | Narrow bandwidth of emotions – often doesn't want to share experiences. Limited emotional vocabulary. |
| Structure and rules | Life chaotic and dramatic. Rebellious, impulsive, breaks the rules. | Tends to follow the rules, likes structure, and also tends to be a 'systematiser'. |
| New experiences | Wants change. Seeking stimulation, novelty, new emotional experiences. | Less open to change or new emotional experiences, although likes new intellectual experiences. |
| Sensory | Occasional aversions to sensory issues, often related to trauma. | Sensory issues are marked, frequently from early childhood (noise, touch etc.). |
| Language | Typical everyday usage. | Can be literal/pedantic, slow at processing, missing 'gist' and humour. |
| Non-verbal | Generally normal. Good at interpreting others, although may overemphasise rejection or criticism cues. | Often poor expressive non-verbal behaviour (eye contact, tone of voice etc.) and understanding of non-verbal behaviours in others. |
| Co-ordination | Normal. | Often clumsy. Motor mannerisms. |
| Self-harm | Usually triggered by sense of interpersonal rejection or being slighted/abused or criticised. Impulsive and not organised. | Triggered by self-criticism, social mistakes, anxiety, guilt and sensory overload. Often methodical dating back to early childhood. |
| Interpersonal directness | Can be indirect. 'Splitting', emotional – blames others. | Very direct, honest. Straightforward, difficulty telling 'white lies'. |

People on the autism spectrum are likely to display compulsions related to hoarding or repetitive ordering, touching or tapping, sexual obsessions or body dysmorphia (feeling that a part of their body is a different shape from normal), whereas individuals with OCD are more likely to have obsessions surrounding cleaning or contamination themes, with compulsions related to counting, washing or checking.

## Eating disorders

Autistic people are at risk of developing eating disorders. It is reported that potentially 20% of people accessing eating disorder services have autism, (Huke et al, 2013; Treasure 2013), albeit many are undiagnosed because of social camouflaging. The presentation of an autistic person in an eating disorder unit is often 'atypical' as it is often less about body image and shape and more about following rules, restricted eating patterns and rigidity concerning certain foods. Individuals with a very restrictive specific eating pattern, where they eat the same food all the time, might get classified as having an eating disorder. Autistic people, particularly high-functioning females, are at very high risk of developing an eating disorder because of the following:

- Focus on the details of food and weight with a perfectionistic eye.

- Once a rule has been learned or accepted, it is difficult to shift.

- Sometimes food and weight can become a 'special fixated interest'.

- Sensory aversions or difficulties with certain foods – e.g. about textures – which makes some food unpalatable.

- An inability to focus on the bigger picture – lack of central coherence.

- Weak ToM or difficulty working out how other people might perceive the person and their weight or body image.

Alice has an atypical eating disorder:

> I don't have a fear of gaining weight but a strict obedience to a set of rules and routines that I depend on for a sense of stability. My focus has always been on a sense of sameness and regulation around numbers, what was and wasn't allowed and when. When I was younger, I always wanted the same number of foods in my lunch or dinner. When I got older it was about counting calories and grams of fat. If I exceeded my allowance I felt like a failure. It wasn't a fear of weight gain or losing weight. I just wanted to stay the same.

## Bipolar disorder

Bipolar disorder is a psychiatric condition previously known as manic depression, characterised by fluctuating and rapidly cycling moods, from elation to despair. A small number of people with autism have comorbid bipolar disorder, but misdiagnosis is common. Many autistic people have a tendency to view the world through rather 'black and white', 'all or nothing', 'good or bad' filters and their mood can very quickly spiral downwards or even upwards. There is not much middle ground in between the extremes. However, it is important not to confuse an autistic person's overexcitement in a special interest with mania, which is qualitatively different in terms of intensity and speed.

## Addiction – substance abuse

It is estimated that between 10 and 20% of people in drugs and alcohol services could be on the autism spectrum. The risk factors are that drugs are a very effective coping strategy for alleviating anxiety, creating a state of relaxation and emotional detachment, a social lubricant, an escape from reality and anaesthetising from past trauma. They also offer membership of a group or subculture of fellow addicts, a 'safe bubble', which does not require extensive communication and provides social acceptance, with clear rules and dress code and a purpose and structure for the day. The process may start with alcohol and marijuana but can escalate into greater dependency and addiction.

## Complex trauma

Autistic people have a much higher incidence of being bullied, abused and traumatised than non-autistic groups. Autistic females are nearly three time more likely to be sexually abused than non-austistic females, possibly because they have trouble understanding social norms or recognizing dangerous situations (Olhsson Gotby et al, 2018). The most prevalent signs are re-experiencing and general hypervigilance or anxiety. However, a comment often made in trauma psychological therapy is that 'if you don't look for it you don't see it'. This certainly seems to be the case in people with autism, where it might be necessary to ask probing questions to elicit exactly what has gone on.

## Gender dysphoria

Gender dysphoria (GD) is not a mental illness; the technical definition is 'distress that accompanies incongruence between an experienced or expressed gender and gender assignment at birth'. People with GD frequently desire to change their appearance and body to be congruent with their gender identity. Research indicates a high incidence of autism in GD clinics; estimates vary between 6 and 26% (Thrower et al, 2020). This is a massive over-representation considering that those with autism represent approximately 1–2% of the population. How to explain this phenomenon?

> Researching into gender issues and testosterone in autism points out that our results suggest that women with ASD have elevated serum testosterone levels and that, in several aspects, they display more masculine traits than women without ASD, and men with ASD display more feminine characteristics than men without ASD. Rather than being a disorder characterized by masculinisation (having male sexual characteristics in a female) in both genders, ASD thus seems to be a gender defiant disorder. Our results strongly suggest that gender incoherence in individuals with ASD is to be expected and should be regarded as one reflection of the wide autism phenotype.
>
> (Bejerot et al, 2012 p.122)

Coleman-Smith (2020) interviewed people with autism in a GD clinic and carried out a thematic analysis. Three main themes emerged: first, 'I felt different from an early age' – one participant commented, 'I never felt I was a girl... I never wanted to wear girl's clothes... I didn't feel I fitted in anywhere'. The second theme was that people generally 'concealed, pushed away and suppressed these gender feelings, which had a negative impact on mental health'. The third theme was that there is a 'percolation of these gender issues', of 'living a lie', which eventually reaches a precipice or some kind of 'critical mass' resulting in an attempt to seek transition.

Sarah Kendrickx in her book, '*Women and Girls with Autism Spectrum Disorder*' (2015), suggested that around 20% of the autistic women that she had spoken to for her book describe themselves as 'asexual', a further 50% define themselves as 'heterosexual'. Kendrickx suggests that many autistic women are more inclined to be 'gender fluid', not feeling either male or female but something else. One client said, 'As a middle-aged woman I do not strongly perceive myself as female. I have often debated whether I am transgender, as I feel I have both traits of the male and female sex but I don't identify with either ... the term gender fluid fits me a lot better'.

Dr Lawson (2019) an autism expert who transitioned from Wendy to Wenn, suggests,

> It does seem likely, for many reasons, that GD is more common in autistic people. When you consider our honesty, our preference for truth and fairness, then gender identity is likely to be more fluid and less binary. Why do we need to fit into a mode of social expectation if we truly don't believe this is who we are? The non-autistic world is governed by social and traditional expectations, but we may not notice these or fail to see them as important. This frees us up to connect more readily with our true gender.

Dr Lawson's point about truthfulness could be linked to the idea that if a person has 'black and white' autistic thinking, they are likely to become single minded and fixated on an idea they find hard to drop. They might find it difficult to appreciate the more flexible concept of a gender spectrum, accepting that gender can be fluid or recognise an 'in-between' 'feminine male'.

It is accepted that autistic people have a poorer sense of self-identity and self-concept, being less confident in their own attributes, potentially due to having poorer autobiographical memories. Wylie (2018) uses his personal experience of name changing to shed potential light on the GD debate. He points out that when autistic individuals adopt aliases or change their names, they are perhaps indicating identity challenges: 'For decades I sensed that I was living in two separate worlds; the realm of "being", integrity and passion and the neurotypical world of obligation and suffering. I changed my name twice to emphasise new chapters of my life… changing names can be extremely empowering'.

## Tips for clients and staff working in a hospital

If an autistic person is admitted to a psychiatric or general hospital, it is likely to be an extremely stressful environment because of sensory issues, unpredictability, lack of routine, communication and social interaction issues. Table 7.3 offers some tips to hospital staff, clients with autism and families.

*Table 7.3* Tips for managing a person with autism in hospital

| Communication | Routines and structure |
|---|---|
| • Keep communication, clear, concise and concrete.<br>• Speak slowly, give small chunks of information.<br>• Be patient. Don't rush the person.<br>• Ask one question at a time.<br>• Minimise options. Instead of 'what would you like to do?' Ask 'which option do you choose: a, b or c?'<br>• Minimise open questions (e.g. how do you feel?) and maximise quantitative measures e.g. Likert scales (rate pain or anxiety out of 10).<br>• Avoid using vague or abstract reference, hypothetical scenarios, metaphor or flippant comments.<br>• Provide visual information (e.g. bullet points) and keep it succinct. Visual timetables, staff photos on noticeboard or rating scales. | • Try to explain what is going to happen, what the processes and routines are. Knowing 'why' something happens in a particular way is important.<br>• Structure, routine and predictability are calming. Have a plan or timetable.<br>• Always keep the patient involved in the process. Maximise joint planning.<br>• Allow the person to maintain routines and any special interests to enhance calmness and engagement.<br>• Allow for plenty of time for aloneness. Too much social interaction can be stressful.<br>• Identify the 'quiet room' or a quiet place on the ward.<br>• Demonstrate and practice at least one method of requesting help, e.g. pressing a call button (label it).<br>• If plans change, let the person know in advance and explain why. |

| Social interaction | Sensory processing differences |
|---|---|
| • Do not interpret reduced eye contact as disinterest or non-engagement.<br>• Avoid casual non-literal language e.g. 'I'll see you in a minute' and then turning up 10 minutes later. Literal and precise is best.<br>• Conversation about special interests will be easier than general social chit-chat that might not come easily.<br>• Check understanding using concept checking questions such as – 'What did we agree?', 'What were the key points discussed?'<br>• Look out for behaviours that might indicate discomfort, pain or distress e.g. agitation, anxiety.<br>• Don't mistake 'bluntness' for rudeness or take it personally.<br>• Involve a carer or family to provide insights into special likes and dislikes.<br>• Be aware that the person might not always understand humour e.g. banter.<br>• Be aware that the patient may not overtly show emotion. | • Autistic people can be over- or under-sensitive to sensory cues. Ask about sensory sensitivities.<br>• Look out for discomfort, distress or distraction caused by environment e.g. lights, noise, smells, temperature, touch or texture.<br>• Consider that individuals with autism may be less attuned to, or able to track and report internal symptoms such as changes in pain or temperature or anxiety.<br>• Pain tolerance may be unusually low or high.<br>• Consider sensory sensitivity when using equipment (e.g. blood pressure cuff) and other procedures (e.g. taking blood).<br>• Let the individual know if you are going to make physical contact, explain what will happen and why, at each step in the process.<br>• Consider environmental adaptions and supports (e.g. noise-cancelling earphones and dimmed lights).<br>• Help make up individual's own sensory comfort pack (headphones, music, sunglasses). |

## Autism and the criminal justice system

The overwhelming majority of autistic people are law-abiding citizens; often with very clear conventional ideas about what is right or wrong. However, young people with autism are more likely than the non-autistic population to enter the criminal justice system, often due to four main types of offending behaviour described in the following sections.

### Problems created by lack of understanding or naïveté

Many autistic individuals find that problems are created by lack of understanding, misinterpretation of social cues, social naivety or immaturity. One scenario might involve inappropriate social behaviours which are interpreted as unwanted sexual advances, or perhaps an inability to identify the age of an individual, could lead to a charge of sexual offences with a minor.

When in custody, autistic individuals are often quick to confess and justify their actions, perhaps not being able to understand what all the fuss is about – they view their actions as logical, justified and appropriate without any associated emotion or remorse. However, there are cases of young women with autism, particularly in residential care, whose social vulnerability has been exploited so that, unfortunately, they have been sexually abused by predatory male staff. Similarly, online, internet interactions can leave vulnerable young autistic women in positions where they are 'groomed', exploited and abused. One mother said,

> Jackie doesn't have a concept of danger; she is much too trusting and is frankly at risk. If she's known somebody online for a week, she thinks they are her new best friend. She has got into cars with men and naively arranged to meet a man in his forties and she is only 17. She will also walk around the streets at night skimpily dressed in the dark. She just doesn't get it!

### Problems arising from disruption to routine

Aggressive behaviour can arise from a disruption to routine, stress from changing a daily routine or from sensory overload. This kind of aggressive behaviour is a reaction of frustration and aggression to a situation of stress or arousal rather than instrumental aggression. Autistic people are often less aware of a gradual build-up of stress and just explode. One man was very sensitive to the noise of a neighbour's dog barking and decided to take the law into his own hands, becoming verbally and physically aggressive towards his neighbour who ended up reporting him to the police. His desire for justice in his problem situation overrode other considerations.

### Problems occurring from preoccupation with a special interest

In some situations, preoccupation with a special interest may lead to an offence. In one case a man with a special interest in tractors stole a tractor that had no practical use and could not have been sold for financial gain. The compulsive nature of the special interest was so strong that the man was tempted to commit an offence without thinking through the consequences.

Two cases of cybercrime have attracted a great deal of press attention over the last decade. Gary McKinnon was a young British man, with Asperger's syndrome, who hacked into the computer system of the US government from his bedroom in his parents' home in North London. He had developed a remarkably high level of computer skill and became obsessed with a special interest in finding out what information the Pentagon kept on its computers. He was socially isolated and showed significant social naivety; he did not comprehend that he had committed a crime or the consequences of his actions; he did not attempt to hide his crime and left notes on each computer saying that he had been there. Gary seemed unable to imagine that the authorities would view his behaviour as criminal or what the social consequences would be. The Americans wanted him extradited and to stand trial for his 'crime' but thankfully the UK authorities recognised that Gary had Asperger's and decided that the threat of prison was a sufficient deterrent to reduce the risk of similar occurrences.

Similarly, Navinder Singh Sarao, a 36-year-old stocks and shares 'trading savant', made $70 million very quickly by rapidly buying and selling financial futures, using a keyboard and mouse, as if playing a computer game, in his parents' spare bedroom in Hounslow. His actions helped precipitate a stock market collapse, the so-called 'flash crash' of 2010, temporarily erasing $1 trillion off the value of stocks. The FBI and US Department of Justice investigated and arrested him for fraud and manipulating the markets and tried to extradite him to the United States. Sarao ended up helping the US government with its investigation and explaining how he had 'tricked' or 'spoofed' the markets.

## Problems associated with vulnerability and court

Autistic individuals are often vulnerable to exploitation by others because they don't understand hidden meanings and intentions. When in custody, they may be more likely to be suggestible and may admit to the crime just so they can remove themselves from the situation. Giving evidence in court can be particularly stressful to those with autism, and using an 'Intermediary' (often a specially trained speech therapist) is desirable. The intermediary's function is to communicate to the vulnerable witness, explain difficult questions and recommend calming measures such as frequent breaks if necessary. They often have to instruct barristers on how to ask questions, avoiding certain language and figures of speech such as 'Bear with me', 'Set me straight', 'Not in any way, shape or form' or 'I'm going to jog your memory'. Many autistic individuals, when cross-questioned, may react very angrily to any insinuation that they have lied and therefore appear more pervasively angry. They may also have extreme difficulty in answering questions which involve having an understanding of what another person's intention is.

## Psychological therapy and adaptations

There are a number of types of psychological therapy for adults on the spectrum that can be very helpful. Immediately after getting a diagnosis, a form of post-diagnostic counselling can be beneficial. This may focus on understanding what autism is, reflecting on how it has affected the person in the past, how it affects the person in the present and planning a future where aspects of autism are accommodated, strengths are optimised and vulnerabilities protected so the authentic, autistic self can flourish. This type of therapy involves helping the person to understand that their brain is wired differently, but is not defective, it's about accepting rather than changing; a journey of unravelling. One man said, 'Diagnosis allows me to live a life attuned to what makes me more comfortable. The therapist is in some ways an "expert companion" on that journey'.

Bulluss and Sesterka (2020) write about the process of having 'support' to assist in the process of correcting inaccurate thoughts, narratives and core beliefs that have developed in the decades prior to receiving a diagnosis. An example of this would be being judged as different and being told 'you are difficult' by an adult neurotypical world in response to undiagnosed autistic traits and behaviour. Support is required to rewrite ideas that have been internalised and unhelpfully become part of their self-concept. Getting a diagnosis offers an explanation and understanding for those behaviours, and the label of 'being difficult' can be reappraised through the lens of autism as being erroneous. One client explained, 'Our diagnosis allowed us a framework by which to break out the red pen and rewrite the narrative of our lives... to confidently strike out the word "difficult" and proudly replace it with "autistic"'. The following examples below show how the word 'difficult', crossed out, can be replaced with the word 'autistic':

- 'I always ask for the same number of ice cubes in my drink because I am ~~difficult~~ autistic'.

- 'I feel overwhelmed at parties because I am ~~difficult~~ autistic'.

- 'I like to talk about topics that interest me rather than small talk because I am ~~difficult~~ autistic'.

- 'I am disconcerted when there are unexpected changes in my environment because I am ~~difficult~~ autistic'.

- 'I need to know specific details in forward planning because I am ~~difficult~~ autistic'.

Psychological therapy post-diagnosis is, amongst other things, about helping and guiding the autistic person to 'unpick' those negative messages, and to modify those behaviours where the autistic person is always trying to 'fit in'. Adapted forms of Cognitive Behavioural Therapy (CBT) and other so-called third-wave types of CBT, specifically, Mentalizing Based Therapy (MBT), known as 'Mindfulness', DBT and Acceptance and Compassion Therapy (ACT), have all been shown useful for treating anxiety, depression or problems with emotional regulation. All approaches might benefit from the adaptations suggested next:

- *Therapist needs to know a bit about autism*: this does not mean they have to be an expert, but they have to have some knowledge, awareness and be interested in the subject.

- *Assess emotional literacy and insight*: it is important to assess and understand the client's initial level of emotional literacy (alexithymia). Does the person struggle to notice physiological changes/sensations in their body (hunger, thirst, pain) or other less obvious sensations that signify emotions such as anxiety, fear, anger and sadness? Can the person correctly label those sensations as emotions and differentiate between emotions, noticing emotional graduations? How easily can the person access their automatic thoughts and discriminate between thoughts, feelings, sensations and behaviour? How able is the person to stand back and reflect on their own thoughts and emotions, 'to be introspective' about what triggers different emotions? How well can the person recognise, for example, what they might do that annoys or upsets another person – to be able to take that other person's perspective.

- *Structure*: adopt a more concrete, explicit, directive, prescriptive structured approach where the context is explained and there is a greater use of written and visual material. Identify treatment goals at the beginning of therapy so the person can have a list of: 'At the end of treatment I would like to have achieved the following goals'. Structure the session with an agenda detailing what you are going to talk about. Write down summaries in bullet points, at the end of sessions.

- *Use visual materials*: autistic people often have difficulty accessing thoughts in a verbal form and tend to be more visual. Use visual materials such as an 'Emotional Thermometer', to rate emotions on a 5-point scale or 'The Emotional Colour Wheel' for recognising emotions (see Appendix 1 page 203). Perhaps use pictures of the body with locations where emotional sensations might be felt or draw diagrams using 'thought bubbles'.

- *Small c and big B*: placing greater emphasis on changing behaviours rather than cognitions - in CBT terms it is small c and big B. Avoid unnecessary introspection and open-ended questions about emotion such as, 'How does that feel?' One client said, 'Helping me understand what I want and how to express it, was much more useful than the years spent trying to understand how I feel'. Another lady at the end of a 6 week 'Being Me' course, (see Appendix 1), when asked what was most useful, commented, 'When one member said that he takes off his glasses in the supermarket so he can't see as well, which means it is less overwhelming to his senses'. However, another client said, 'Everything I know about my emotions and those of other people I've learned in the five years of counselling that I've had since I was 15. It never came intuitively to me, it's all learned'.

- *Use plain language*: using plain English and avoiding the use of metaphors, ambiguity and hypothetical situations. Keep it concrete and literal. Use the client's own words to describe symptoms.

- *Be specific and direct*: try to avoid broad vague open-ended questions or comments that might be misconstrued like, 'How does that sound?' Keep it clear, simple, practical, ask more directive questions, rather than indirect/reflective so-called Socratic questions.

- *Set rules for communication*: autistic clients have social communication difficulties. This means that therapy will need to include rules as to when the therapist can interrupt (if the client is verbose), and how the client will indicate that they don't understand something (if they are passive and unlikely to say so).

- *Suggest alternatives*: because of difficulty in cognitive flexibility and poor imagination to generate new ideas, deliberately suggest specific alternatives. A forced-choice question, where you give the person a number of options, or a dropdown list can be helpful, e.g. 'when is the problem worse in the supermarket or at home? Rather than a, 'what do you think?' type of interventions. Avoid 'meaningful silences'. It is also important to check whether the person has understood. You might also have to slow down.

- *Environment*: using the same therapy room helps so the person doesn't have to process information again and again. Be aware of sensory sensitivities like bright lights, external noise, wearing strong aftershave/ perfume or the presence of a ticking clock, which can all be distracting. If the person has a slow processing speed, it might mean having shorter sessions, offering breaks, or even offering longer sessions – check it out. For some people, going out for a walk to talk can be preferable to sitting in two chairs facing each other.

- *Include psycho-educational material and skills training*: educational material about emotional awareness, bodily physiological sensations, identifying triggers to emotions and unravelling what is related to autism and what might be something else like depression or camouflaging is useful. Teaching social and coping skills and safety behaviours is necessary, contrary to strict CBT guidelines, because the autistic person may have significant skills deficits, particularly regarding social anxiety.

- *Involve others*: involving a family member, partner, carers or professionals can have benefits if the person agrees. This might ease anxiety, help to share knowledge and be an aid for the person to remember and understand the key points. I remember having a client's 'best friend' in the session who would often say, 'she hasn't understood what you've just said, I can tell. She nods her head and pretends she understands but she doesn't'.

• *Be creative*: it is important to be flexible and creative in order to maintain the person's attention. Incorporating their special interest in the therapy, if possible, can be helpful. So for example, having a 10-point rating scale of emotions and moods based on a favourite interest, for example, Harry Potter characters, with Harry as 0, Professor Trelawney as 5 and Voldemort as 10. Another man whose interest was HiFi conceptualised his emotions by depicting the bars of a graphic equaliser.

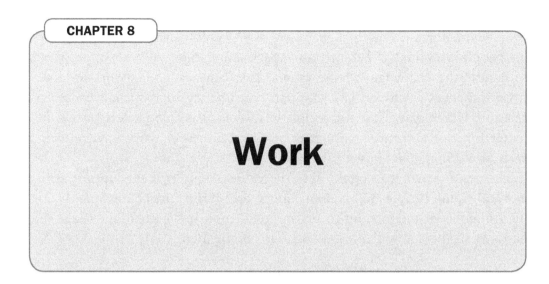

# CHAPTER 8

# Work

## An underused employment resource

Employment is the glue which holds most people's lives together; it provides structure, routine, purpose and meaning. One might think that as we live in a digital age, autism would 'fit' well into the digital workforce. But unfortunately unemployment rates are high among autistic people, even when compared with other disability groups. In the United Kingdom, the percentage of autistic adults in full-time employment is estimated to be about 16% and only 32% are in any paid work at all, although three quarters want to work; the proportion of unemployed graduates with autism is approximately 26% (National Autistic Society, 2016). Autistic people have the potential to be good workers, liking to have a project, a routine, a structure, something to get on with; they are conscientious, hardworking, preferring not to spend time chatting, socialising or gossiping. The present situation undoubtedly highlights a waste of a good resource. A further positive aspect is that if autistic people can be accommodated within a job, they tend to stay, and having a stable workforce, with good retention, is highly beneficial for any company. One man, who is a researcher at a university, commented, 'I don't want to move from this job unless I'm forced to. I'm happy to do it for the rest of my life; even when I retire I'll probably still keep coming to the campus as a volunteer'.

There is a growing realisation of the benefits of having a neurodiverse workforce, because autistic people think differently, make connections that others do not, are innovative and solve problems. Some large companies have sought out or positively discriminated in favour of people with autism, such as Goldman Sachs and Microsoft. One Danish company called The Specialists, which tested electronic equipment, computer programs and new telephone systems, was managed by a man, with child, who actively sought out employees with autism because of their eye for detail and enjoyment of repetitive tasks. German software giant SAP hopes to recruit hundreds of people with autism. The chief executive of SAP comments, 'Only by employing people who think differently and spark innovation will SAP be prepared to handle the challenges of the twenty-first century ... innovation comes from the edges'. Auticon is a German consultancy that opened offices in London, which places autistic people in IT companies and offers staff a different form of autism friendly interview and an easier work environment, such as working from home.

There is a growing recognition of the value of employment support agencies in helping people with autism find work, write curriculum vitae, cope with interviews and explain to prospective employers something about the needs of the person with autism. Belinda commented,

> I've struggled with bullying at work before, but now I've got a diagnosis, a new job and a good boss. He has contacted Access to Work (the Employment Support Agency) and they have provided me with a job coach, who is really helpful. She is going to deliver to colleagues and other managers training in 'Working with Autism and Neurodiversity'.

One 'silver lining' from the Covid-19 lockdown, when many people were asked to work from home, was that it suited many autistic people. John commented,

> I love working from home. No more idle chat around the coffee machine, no more office politics, no more genuflecting to the boss every time you see him or her, no more trying to find a hide-away. Given the right IT skill set, working from home should be ideal for many 'Aspies'.

## Reasonable adjustments

If an autistic person discloses their diagnosis at work (see Chapter 9, p177–180), the company has a legal obligation to make 'reasonable adjustments'. This is because having a diagnosis of autism qualifies as a disability under the Equalities Act (2010). The employer is duty bound to consider making 'reasonable adjustments' to the working environment, if they are practical, can be implemented, can be afforded, will be effective in reducing the disadvantage of the disabled person and they do not have an adverse effect on the health and safety of others. Below are some examples:

- 'We employ a hot desk system, which really stresses me out, because I struggle to handle the change. My manager knows my diagnosis and allowed me to have a fixed desk by the window, in a corner location, with a wall behind me, so it's not too busy'.

- 'I work in an open plan office and don't like being interrupted. I have been allowed to have a model of a set of traffic lights on my desk. If it's on red it means "stop if you are thinking of interrupting me", amber is "only interrupt if it's important" and green mean "go on, it's okay to speak to me". Amazingly it works well'.

- 'We don't have the radio on all the time at work now and they have dimmed the lights, which has really helped me'.

- 'My manager allows me to wear noise cancelling headphones at work so I am not distracted by background noise'.

- 'My manager has made a point of always having an agenda and minutes for meetings, circulated at least three days in advance, because he knows that for me a meeting without an agenda stresses me out. I need to be prepared'.

- 'I am allowed to work at home 2 days a week, which means I can cope better with 3 days in the office'.

- 'I am permitted a break after meetings, which I find exhausting. I have been allowed to take a respite and go for a 15-minute walk in the nearby park, which I find very soothing'.

- 'My manager always checks out my understanding of a task and writes it down for me in a very specific language, with bullet points, because without that I can easily misunderstand what I'm requested to do'.

- 'I have a mentor at work, who "keeps an eye on me" – I talk to him if there are any problems. It's very helpful as he can smooth things over particularly if I've been a bit too blunt'.

- 'I have been allocated a "buddy" within the office who supported me to attend the Christmas party and helped me find ways to deal with small talk and discuss other topics rather than just my special interests'.

- 'I'm allowed reduced face-to-face contact with clients, largely because when I see them I make an effort to camouflage which is very tiring'.

- 'My manager has arranged autism awareness training for those that work with me'.

## Know your strengths and weaknesses

For an autistic person, or for anybody, having good insight and understanding into how their particular brain works is a helpful factor in being successful in employment. It is important to understand your strengths and weaknesses and to anticipate the situations that are going to be challenging. There are many advantages that an autistic person might have in the workplace and these need to be highlighted. Nick comments, 'When I focus on writing a programme I forget to eat, drink and go to the bathroom; I'm so engrossed. All I need is a computer and a bed'. In contrast, typical weakness are often poor 'executive functioning', including skills such as being able to stand back and 'see the big picture', to plan and organise, and multitask and prolonged face-to-face interaction, which requires good social skills. In an ideal world, a vocational assessment with an independent professional would be good, but finding an occupational psychologist with a good knowledge of autism is not easy. So the assessment might have to be done with a close family member or friend or by making an accurate appraisal by metaphorically looking in the mirror. A good exercise is for the person to sit down with somebody who knows them well and draw up a list of strengths and challenges.

Below is a list of potentially positive qualities of people with autism in the workplace and then a list of less positive qualities or challenges – but everybody is different. A useful exercise is to go through the list, either alone or with somebody and identify which apply.

Strengths/positive qualities:

- Reliable and hard-working – conscientious wants to 'do a good job'.

- Perfectionistic – likes to 'get it right', accurate, good at identifying errors, eye for detail.

- Persistent – likes to finish a job – tenacity, keeps going however long it takes.

- Logical, analytical and numerical – technically very able – knowledgeable, methodical, good with systems.

- Honest – likes to stick to the rules – strict moral code, doesn't cut corners.

- Thrives on routine and clear expectations. Likes to have a fixed ordered plan. Doesn't get bored with routine or repetition.

- Doesn't waste time chatting, socialising or bothering with 'office politics' – prefers to get on with the job.

- Happy to work independently.

- Loyal and committed. If the person likes the work, he or she is likely to stick with it. Unlikely to be searching for new experiences or fresh challenges.

- Special skills: good at absorbing and retaining facts, often has in-depth knowledge about particular subjects, and novel and innovative solutions to problem solving.

Weaknesses/challenges:

- Teamwork skills often poor – not good at fitting in with a group and socialising.

- Communication of own needs is often poor – not very good at recognising stress, communicating own needs and asking for help.

- When stressed potential for emotional breakdown or 'meltdowns'.

- Conflict resolution sometimes poor – can fall out with people by being too honest or blunt, or due to rather rigid views and intolerances.

- Poor executive skills, poor organisation and planning, poor at juggling multiple tasks, switching attention, prioritising, making decisions.

- Misinterpreting instructions – needs clear unambiguous instructions and sometimes others to check out that message is understood.

- Coping with change poor – needs plenty of warning and preparation for change.

- Management of others can be problematic – due to not recognising the needs of others, lack of flexibility and difficulty resolving conflict.

- Possible unconventional habits and manners may make more vulnerable to teasing.

- Very sensitive to the sensory environment, so that background noise, light, smells, temperature may be more of a problem than for the non-autistic person.

## Turning a special interest into a career

Autistic people often have all encompassing, strong special interests, in which they have accumulated vast pools of specialist knowledge, skill and expertise. Why not attempt to use that interest to develop a career? Universities are full of people with special interests who are paid to talk about their subjects. Here are three examples of clients who have used their special interest to build a career.

*Farook* works as a translator for a large broadcasting company:

> I was born in a poor village in Sudan, and both my parents were illiterate. At school I was always top of my class but socially I didn't interact well and was bullied. I was not particularly popular at school because I used to correct the teachers, was opinionated, awkward and poor at sports. I spent most of my childhood reading, especially newspapers, and listening to news bulletins. From a very early age I knew all the members of the political Cabinet and the capitals of all the countries in the world and studied Arabic poetry, being able to remember hundreds of lines of poetry quite easily. I eventually went to the university in Khartoum where I studied English language and enjoyed translation work. I came to the UK in 2001 applying for political asylum and eventually obtained a job as a translator and Middle East expert and media analyst for a large broadcasting organization. I became so passionate about translating that I spent hours and hours after work

doing translation work. Translating is my passion – I would do it for free. I almost can't believe people are paying me to do this.

*Fay* who works as a museum curator has a similar feeling about her job:

> At secondary school people used to think I was rather odd as I hated sport and was not interested in pop music or make-up. I was interested in Sir Francis Drake and the Elizabethans and then slightly later, the Egyptians and the Druids. I studied archaeology at university and eventually became a museum curator. I had to pinch myself the other day when I was cataloguing Roman pottery and I realised I was doing something I really enjoyed and was being paid for it.

*Marie* is a lawyer who specialises in family law and commented:

> As a 12-year-old I remember going to my local magistrate and Crown Court and sitting in the visitors' gallery being fascinated by the proceedings. The law became something of an obsession to me. I'm now working as a solicitor specialising in family law. I still struggle with the people, and my eye contact is not good, but once a client gets to know me they know I know my business and will do the best for them.

## Challenge (i): Getting through the job interview

The recruitment process is a problem for a number of reasons; application forms may be unclear, with abstract questions and the interview itself is often a test of social ability, rather than the ability to do the job, which can disadvantage the autistic person. There is growing recognition of the value of employment support agencies, or advocates, in helping people with autism find and keep a job.

For most jobs, there is an interview process which can be problematic. One man said,

> I'm bad at interviews because I can't explain myself or answer questions on the spot – I need time. I find it difficult to understand the nuance of the questions when the questions have several meanings. I think my autism affects my ability to give a good first impression at interview – I come across as awkward. In fact my last boss said, 'I really wasn't sure about you at the interview but you've turned out really well'. I also think that a major problem these days is that the pendulum has swung too far in the direction of 'must be a good team player'.

Wylie (2015) reports that he has had some success with the unusual strategy of when applying for a job, to volunteer his services free of charge for a few days before the interview. In that way, employers became more aware of his skills and abilities to compensate for his awkward performance at the interview.

*Tips*:

- Read the job description beforehand and reflect back an understanding of the job.

- Ask clarifying questions to make sure you have correctly interpreted what is being said.

- A few ready prepared questions to ask at the end of the interview are also sensible as invariably the interviewee will be asked, 'Do you have any questions?'

- Practice beforehand, maybe role playing with a trusted person firing questions at the interviewee.

- It is also sensible for the person being interviewed to make a list of behaviours they should and shouldn't do. Examples might be, make appropriate greeting, make good eye contact and don't bite nails.

- Consider some soft disclosure, where there is an acknowledgement that there is a difference between being good at an interview and doing the job itself.

## Challenge (ii): Social demands

A job is often not just the person's ability to do the job, but the social and interpersonal side of work, communication between the person and their manager and colleagues. One man said, 'It almost feels like I have two jobs simultaneously rather than one. One is doing my work, which I enjoy and am good at; the other is expending huge amounts of energy on maintaining a social interface'. Another lady commented about the general stresses in her job just before Christmas:

> I'm only doing a small clerical job at the university and sometimes think, 'What is the point?'. I've told them I'm not going to the Christmas party, but this week there was a leaving lunch for somebody and my work colleagues laid out all the food on my desk! Then somebody has thought up this idea of having a cocktail competition, where we're all put in teams. I don't want to be involved. I'm there to work.

*Tips*:

- Try to strike a balance between assertively saying 'no' to social events and compromising and joining in some events for a limited time. Maybe say, 'I'll come for an hour'.

- If appropriate, disclose reasons to key colleagues and ask for help. Identifying one person – a buddy – and ask for help with for example managing 'small talk'.

## Challenge (iii): Being successful, getting promoted – the 'halo effect'

The 'halo effect' is a common scenario within the business world, that is, if a person is good at one particular job, people assume that they will be brilliant with everything, resulting in the person being promoted to being a manager. But managing other people is a completely different skill set from 'doing the job'. Ashley Stanford's book, *Business for 'Aspies'* (2011), is based on her experience of working with her husband Michael, who has an autism diagnosis and is an exceptionally gifted technical programmer. Together the couple have successfully developed an IT company in the Silicon Valley area of the United States. She tells the story of how Michael, earlier in his career, was promoted to manage others because he was such a great programmer and technical problem solver. His limited time as a manager always ended in disaster because he just wanted to be left alone to write good code; he had difficulty 'putting himself in others' shoes' and empathising with and understanding the needs of others when they were different from his own. Stanford describes in her book the environment she has had to create for her husband to work at his optimal level. An overriding message of the book is, 'Focus on the positives and the negatives disappear'. However, in this situation, the moral is that the brightest and most able person is often not the best manager.

Success also brings rewards that sometimes might be stressful and challenging. In the United Kingdom, singer Susan Boyle won a TV talent show, and her records began selling in millions – success changed her life as she became a celebrity. The demands of coping with appearing on TV chat shows, being interviewed by journalists, photographed by the paparazzi and having her private life scrutinised were a very different skill set from singing a song in tune. Susan had undiagnosed Asperger's and initially struggled to cope.

Rebecca, a research scientist at a university, was investigating climate change and cloud formations and made a research breakthrough. She had an article published in the prestigious journal *Nature* which transformed her life. She commented,

> Overnight I became something of a celebrity, having my photograph in the newspaper, being interviewed on television and by the press and being invited to champagne receptions at various universities. I found these social functions extremely stressful as I was happiest on my own, sitting at my desk, quietly analysing the data. I became increasingly anxious and stressed until I had a 'nervous breakdown' and made a suicide attempt. I was referred to a Community Mental Health Team, who mistakenly diagnosed borderline personality disorder. After over a year of medication and not very helpful psychological therapy, I was diagnosed as having Asperger's syndrome. It was like someone had turned the lights on.

*Tips*:

- Recognise your strengths and weaknesses. Good technicians might not make good managers, requiring different skill sets.

- Think about the skills required to be a good manager and decide whether you have those skills. If success has catapulted you into a different more 'social world', you need to negotiate it carefully, protecting yourself.

- Talk it over with somebody who will give you good feedback, stay grounded and attempt to carry on doing, or stay in contact with, the original task that brought success.

## Challenge (iv): Dealing with sudden unexpected change

People with autism thrive on routine, sameness, predictability, repeatability and knowing what is coming next.

Variety is not necessarily the spice of life, and the emotion of surprises is often the equivalent of terror. People often say they are physically ill preparing for change. Jim had worked for the post office for 20 years sorting the mail and his story is relevant.

> I'd studied history at university, but enjoyed the sorting job because it gave me an income, a regular rhythm and routine and I could listen to my audio tapes on the history of the First and Second World Wars while I worked. I had my own sorting frame with different compartments for different postcodes and areas and was the quickest sorter of mail in the south east of England. One Monday morning I came in and my sorting frame had been moved. A new management team decided that they wanted to implement some changes and decided to move me to work on a different area and take on more responsibility. I was absolutely furious and had a real 'meltdown' with the new manager, pinning him against a wall. I was suspended, had a breakdown, resulting in nine months off work. I saw a psychiatrist for depression, and then got a referral to a psychologist who diagnosed Asperger's syndrome. I did manage to successfully return to work but not before all managers within the sorting office were given autism awareness training.

Sally had worked at an animal and canine rehabilitation centre for 10 years and according to her boss, was, '*amazingly good with the animals and at her job*'. However, Sally was quiet; not very verbal, found it difficult to express herself or communicate and recently had gone off work with 'depression'; friends and work colleagues couldn't understand what was wrong. Sally didn't at the time have a diagnosis of autism, but the treating psychiatrist suspected it and made a referral. Sally was clearly autistic, a diagnosis was made and the roots of the problem explored and identified. It appears that recent changes at work have been particularly stressful as there were more new people on her shift and the environment was much noisier. The work area had become the same place as the break area so that Sally had nowhere to go to get away from people. A treadmill, which was noisy, was introduced and she could hear a radio in a different room. Sally was a person who had rather rigid routines for her work practice as well as significant sensory issues around noise. She had a quiet breakdown and couldn't communicate what the problems were, partly because she wasn't fully aware of them herself. Once the situation was recognised, management made a huge effort to accommodate Sally and get her back to work, not just because she was so good at her job, but also because she was so well liked.

*Tips*:

• Alert managers that sudden change is particularly stressful and it needs to be gradual and thought through.

• Talk it through with a friend or colleague, identifying the difficulties, ways of coping and benefits.

## Challenge (v): 'Reading between the lines' – misinterpreting communication

Reading between the lines, or interpreting complex information that might be ambiguous, is sometimes a problem. Alan had worked for the Ministry of Defence on an army base for 15 years as a warehouseman and delivery driver. He was conscientious and really enjoyed his job, although he wasn't very sociable and had a number of 'run-ins' and fallouts with people and was known as being 'a little odd or eccentric'. He usually arrived at work between 07.40 and 08.00 every morning and often worked over his allotted hours or through his lunch break so that he got the job done. A number of influential friendly colleagues had always said, 'It doesn't matter exactly what time you get in as long as the job is done'. The Ministry of Defence then launched an initiative called 'Flexible Working Hours Policy', which came in a four-page document, with complicated language, multiple clauses and small print. Computerised time sheets were also introduced. Alan signed the document, without fully understanding it, thinking that he was agreeing to carry on working 'flexibly'. A senior manager had even commented, 'just carry on with the flexi'. However, although the document was entitled 'Flexible Working Hours Policy', what it really meant was the opposite. Employees were given a choice of a number of shifts and then had to stick to those shifts. Alan had signed the form for the shift that expected employees to arrive at 07.30 and work until 04.00. But because the document was entitled 'Flexible Working Hours Policy', Alan took the meaning literally and carried on as previously getting in at between 07.30 and 07.50 and working after 04.00 to complete a job if it was required. Alan had moved from one department to another and didn't have a settled line manager and nobody had spelt out to him what he needed to do and what he was doing was wrong. Because he was rather isolated and didn't mix with his co-workers at breaks and lunchtime, he didn't get the feedback and information that might have occurred in casual chit-chat. Unfortunately, Alan was disciplined and was suspended. At the time Alan didn't have a diagnosis of autism and only received one a year later after he had collapsed into depression.

*Tips*:

- Seek help in understanding complex ambiguous legal, health and safety and policy communications from a trustworthy person. Check out the meaning. Ask, 'Have I missed something here?'.

- Ask your manager to always check out understanding and write down instructions clearly and literally in bullet points.

## Challenge (vi): Being too honest and upsetting others

Autistic people often say what they think in a very honest, direct, blunt manner, without always considering the emotional impact on the listener. This can often create problems in the workplace. Ceara was a senior nurse, married with children, who had worked in the paediatric intensive care unit of a large teaching hospital for 20 years and had undiagnosed autism. She commented,

> I've always been really good with the technical stuff, medical information, and medications – better than most of the doctors. I don't get attached to patients and just get on with it. I'm a bit robotic in my dealings with patients and their relatives, but I have recently learned to say, 'I'm sorry' to a relative if a baby dies. My communication difficulties have always been brought up in appraisals. I recently got suspended from work for apparently bullying another member of staff, but I wasn't bullying her. I was just telling her what she had done wrong, so she wouldn't make the same mistake next time. I suppose I might have been a bit blunt or outspoken and didn't really take into account that she was upset after the little baby had died. After I got the diagnosis and went back to work I told my colleagues and asked them for more direct feedback, saying, 'tell me if I'm being too blunt or if I've upset you. I can't tell and there is no intention'. Most colleagues responded well, particularly the young ones'.

*Tips*:

- Ask for feedback from a trusted colleague or identify somebody at work as a mentor or buddy.

- Tell people that you can't help being honest and direct and that your judgement of when this is appropriate is suspect and you might need help. Give people permission saying, 'tell me if I'm being a bit direct or too blunt'.

## Challenge (vii): Sensory overload

Work environments can pose all kinds of stresses in terms of assaulting our senses, particularly with noise, light and smell. Flickering neon lights, noisy open plan offices, groups of people chatting, people with strong scent or aftershave are recognised problems. If stress levels are already high, such additions can easily tip people over the edge. Eden worked in an office and made the following comments,

> They moved some other people into the open plan office and one had a really noisy computer, which really affected my concentration. We called IT in and they found that it was vibrating on the desk, so we put padding underneath. Another woman was constantly jiggling her feet behind me and I could feel the vibrations on the floor – it drives me mad! Then they interviewed a lady for a job who smelt of really strong perfume – a melange of odours. I felt like saying please don't employ that person. It's the social side and sensory side of the job which make me feel stressed. The job itself is a doddle.

*Tips*:

- Identify what the triggers are for your sensory overload, e.g. noise and light. See if the environment can be adapted and try to create the optimal environment to work in. Reasonable adjustments might include a seat by the window, or to wear noise cancelling headphones, or even to work at home occasionally. See Chapter 5 on managing sensory sensitivities.

- Make sure you are as comfortable as possible and that your level of sensory discomfort is as low as possible. Then when random sensory challenges come along, you have some existing capacity to cope.

## Challenge (viii): Overload and 'meltdowns'

Overwhelming sensory input from lights, noise and smells combined with multiple mental and social demands often lead to overload, ensuing internal panic and 'meltdowns'. Often it is a build-up of little things over the course of a day and then a final straw that leads to a loss of internal stability and a downwards spiral. Autistic people often don't have a very good gauge to filter how much stress is piling up, and end up crashing after the stress becomes too much. It is crucial that we recognise overload and its consequences. Meltdowns are an example of the fight-or-flight-freeze response – either an angry outburst, or running away or playing dead and being passive. People end up getting angry or anxious and saying or doing things they regret, losing relationships and jobs.

Richard commented as follows:

> I lost my previous job because I had a meltdown – I got angry with a colleague. My manager at the time said it was the last straw even though I was doing the job better than anyone else. In my present job I have 'come out' and told my manager I have Asperger's and can occasionally lose it and become an inarticulate spluttering angry person. What I said is 'Please don't take it personally – it's not personal'. It's the situation that makes me so frustrated that my 'inner switch' is flipped – I'm a bit like Jekyll and Hyde – I can't escape from the monster in me. Usually I need to retire to a quiet place where I can be alone for a while so I can decompress and wait for the inner switch to flip back to the calm mode.

Carol commented as follows:

> Sometimes I have to just get out – but there is nowhere private as my office is all open plan and the building I work in just has glass offices. I either go for a walk in my heavy coat with a big hood or I go to my car in the underground car park. I keep a sleeping bag and can curl up on the back seat pulling the bag over my head for 10 minutes. Then I feel recharged and better able to cope.

*Tips*:

- Be proactive rather than reactive. Try to anticipate stress build-up and identify what the triggers might be.

- Have a strategy such as: leaving the situation, retreating to a calm environment before a meltdown occurs. Better to walk out and say, 'You will have to excuse me', than stay and damage delicate relationships.

- Afterwards apologise and maybe partially explain. Tell people.

## Challenge (ix): 'Whistle blowing'

Many autistic people are scrupulously honest and have a very strong sense of what is, 'right and wrong', which means it is difficult to ignore or turn a blind eye to someone behaving dishonestly at work. Penny worked at a large local leisure centre as a sports officer, really enjoying her job, but ended up leaving after she became a 'whistle blower'. All this happened before she obtained her diagnosis. Penny comments,

> I enjoyed my job but was never any good at mixing with people, or 'banter' with others and could never pick up when people were joking. I liked to get on with the job, follow the rules and get things right. I was really upset by some of the practices of some of the older members of staff which included allowing friends and family to enroll their children free of charge on certain courses and on one occasion selling old equipment such as table tennis tables and not giving the money back to the council. I just couldn't let it go. I have an absolute sense of right and wrong, always follow the rules and would never even walk on the grass if it said not to. I reported it to my manager, which created all sorts of problems as afterwards I was bullied and teased and then when I reported another member of staff for bullying, he said he was joking. Then it seemed all relationships got worse. I couldn't work out who was supportive of me or who was against me and couldn't resolve all the conflicts and became depressed and eventually left.

Penny's difficulty reading people's intentions and understanding their perspectives, honesty, rigid moral code and difficulty managing conflict, all contributed to her losing a job she loved.

*Tips*:

- If a misdemeanour is noticed at work, rather than reporting it straight away, it might be valuable to discuss and weigh up the pros and cons of such a course of action, with a trusted friend or work mentor.

- Consider the advantages of saying nothing and 'letting it go'.

## Challenge (x): Managing eye contact and other non-verbal behaviours

To survive in the work arena, there is often a need to try to improve or at least conceal poor eye contact. The eyes are a powerful communication tool and, without intending, can cause people with autism serious problems at work. Because of poor eye contact, you might be accused of being 'shifty'; conversely, staring eye contact might lead to claims of sexual harassment. An assertive step is to tell colleagues at work that you have difficulties with eye contact and reading people's facial expression, by saying something like,

> I'm sorry but I do not read faces as well as most people do. Could you explain what you mean in words rather than showing me via your face? Alternatively, 'I'm sorry if my eye contact is poor but I have a sensory integration disorder and find it difficult to look at

someone and listen to them at the same time. I am listening to every word you say even though I'm not looking'.

If eye contact is a major personal problem, it might be best to focus on jobs that have less face time or are often more flexible where you either work on your own, or from home.

*Tips*:

- Look near their eyes, maybe at their forehead or upper lip rather than directly in the other person's eyes.

- Glance away often, but when the other person looks away take the opportunity to look at their face. Allow your eyes to glaze over – allow your eyes to relax.

- Tell people that you have a problem.

- Work in a job with limited face-to-face time.

## Challenge (X1): Reaching a point where disclosure is necessary

James was a surgeon in a large teaching hospital, diagnosed with autism five years previously, who chose not to fully disclose his diagnosis to his work colleagues. His reasoning was,'I don't want my diagnosis to define me'. Unfortunately, James became involved in a number or grievances, complaints and a disciplinary hearing, one of which was for 'bullying and harassment', all involving other members of staff. He was accused of 'not being a team player'. There had never been a complaint from his patients and by all accounts he was an excellent practitioner. He was suffering from depression and becoming increasingly isolated form his team. Reasonable allowances had been implemented where any minutes or agendas for meetings were distributed three days beforehand and most of his communication was online rather than face to face. The situation reached a point where James felt that he was on the verge of dismissal, so he disclosed his diagnosis to his immediate manager and the medical director. Both reported "it was like a lightbulb moment, suddenly it explained everything. Previously we thought he was just being awkward". The hospital managers arranged a training session with an autism specialist, inviting 40 of his senior colleagues with the rationale: "James is struggling and there are people out there who genuinely want to help".

*Tips*:

- It would have been helpful if James had disclosed his diagnosis earlier when he had received the first disciplinary.

- It would have helped if a nominated colleague was appointed as a mentor/advocate/support.

## Different thinking styles for different jobs

Temple Grandin in her book *The Autistic Brain* (2014) makes some interesting suggestions about how there are different types of autistic brains, which determine the person's particular skill, and therefore the type of job that they might be best at. She had previously written a bestselling book entitled *Thinking in Pictures* which describes how she had visualised humane livestock-handling facilities, in which she had visualised how frightening it was for a cow to be herded onto a channel with a sharp turn, almost as a film in her head. She points out that she was the visual thinker and thought of the concepts such as the layout of the plant – the slaughter house, the packaging floor and so on, but she required somebody else, a 'pattern thinker', the qualified engineer, who calculated the roof trusses, the spacing and the concrete specifications. Grandin initially made the assumption that the majority of autistic people think in pictures like her, until confronted by a member of her audience at a presentation who disagreed. Grandin now suggests that there are three overlapping systems of thinking: visual or picture thinkers, verbal thinkers and a new category called pattern thinkers.

| *Jobs for picture thinkers* | *Jobs for word fact thinkers* |
|---|---|
| • Architect | • Translator |
| • Photographer | • Librarian/archivist |
| • Graphic artist | • Copy editor/proofreader |
| • Web designer | • Accountant |
| • Computer troubleshooter | • Book and record keeper |
| • Landscape gardener | • Technical writer |
| • Satellite map analyst | • Translator |
| • Plumber | • Data analyst |
| • Engineer | • Speech therapist |
| • Computer animator | • Information officer |
| • Technician | • Writer |
| • Cartographer | • University lecturer/researcher |
| • Artist | • Policy writer |
| • Actor | • Database manager |
| | • Secretary/typist/administrator |

| *Jobs for pattern thinkers* | *Jobs with structure and limited face time* |
|---|---|
| • Computer programmer | • Cleaner |
| • Engineer | • Gardener |
| • Physicist | • Drivers – coach/taxi/bus/lorry |
| • Music composer | • Assembly line worker |
| • Statistician/mathematician | • Craftsperson |
| • Chemist | • Horticulturalist |
| • Scientific researcher | • Safety/security officer |
| • Actuary | • Postman and post woman |
| • Mathematical/financial analyst | • Animal trainer/worker |
| • Music or math's teacher | • Delivery person |
| • Electrician | • Milkman or milk woman |
| • Movement/dance notary | • Warehouse/storeperson |
| • Cyber security | • Night shift worker |

Different thinkers complement each other. Grandin says that she co-authored the book *The Autistic Brain* with a man called Richard Panek and commented how well they worked as a team. She was a picture thinker and visualised the main ideas and the overall picture, and he was a pattern thinker, picking out the patterns, structuring and organising the book.

## Tips for managing an autistic person

Here are a number of simple tips that might be helpful for managers working with individuals on the autism spectrum.

- *Explain tasks clearly*: try to be specific, avoiding the abstract vague and hypothetical and possibly supplement spoken instructions with written bullet pointed instructions.

- *One task at a time*: it is best to deal with and focus on one task at a time, rather than giving multiple tasks at the same time.

- *Avoid ambiguous language – be specific*: try to avoid ambiguous open-ended questions. For example, 'Tell me about yourself' is very vague and the person may not be able to judge what information to give.

- *Be aware that language may be interpreted literally*: asking 'How did you find your last job?' may result in 'I saw an advert in the paper'.

- *Check it out*: ask if the autistic person has understood and give regular feedback about their performance. If they are talking too much let them know and give feedback, as they may find it hard to judge.

- *Communication difficulties are unintentional*: being too honest, which comes across as being blunt or rude and saying the 'wrong' thing, is probably unintentional. Try not to take it personally. Remind other colleagues where appropriate.

- *Socialising difficulties*: being socially awkward, difficulty with small talk, socialising, networking and making friends is common. Allowances need to be made. Identify a work place buddy to help the autistic person negotiate social events at work.

- *Try to find causes of their anxiety*: the person with autism is probably not very good at identifying what is stressing them and then might struggle to articulate this – try to find out in a one-to-one session.

- *Don't take it personally*: being blunt, brutally honest, failing to take into account the feelings of others and having 'meltdowns' is not uncommon. Try not to take it personally as there is probably 'no malice aforethought'.

- *Be aware of change*: sameness, routine and predictability are core desirabilities in autism. If change is needed, gradually prepare the person for it.

- *Be aware of sensory issues – prepare the environment*: sensitivity to noise, light, smells, touch or temperature and difficulty filtering things out can be easily 'overloaded' and might be an issue. A seat by the window might help.

## Tips for autistic people to cope with work

- *Make time for yourself*: when presented with somebody asking for a decision and you are not ready, practice the pre-scripted response of saying, 'Can I get back to you later in the day?'. Give yourself time to consider a reasonable response.

- *Try to keep brain space*: keep brain space and self-protect against overload by focusing on one thing at a time. Ignore the rest. If you are a hyperfocuser, your brain doesn't want to be seeing too many things to do at once.

- *Control your working environment*: try wearing headphones when working to block out noise distraction, have your favourite soundtrack on your headphones that can help you calm down, dim the lights on your desk, have a drawer full of fidget toys, things you can play with like a Rubik's cube.

- *Learn to say 'no' and prioritise*: this is a key assertiveness skill in any walk of life. We all have only a limited capacity and it is important to work out what to prioritise and what to say 'no' to. This is easier said than done and is an area where you might have to ask for help from a job coach, manager, mentor, work buddy or friend.

- *Asking for help*: this is often a good idea as it shows you are engaged in team work. Tell people you might not always be able to interpret their facial expression or moods and might need a few extra clues.

- *Have somewhere to escape to*: one useful strategy is to find a safe place to escape to when things become too overwhelming, e.g. the quiet room, bathroom or park bench.

## A sample letter to employers

Often after a diagnostic assessment the client ends up with a lengthy, detailed report, often with considerable personal information, that is unsuitable for employers. Below is an example of a brief standardised letter for employers which might be helpful.

To Whom It May Concern
Re: Daniel Smith DOB
Daniel was assessed on (date) at the Adult Autism Assessment Service.

His developmental history and profile of abilities meets criteria for a diagnosis of Autism. In the workplace, this means that Daniel brings a range of distinct positives. Those with Autism tend to be,

- Reliable and hard working.

- Persistent, in that they are highly motivated to finish a job.

- Perfectionistic and likes to 'get it right', are highly motivated to be accurate, are good at identifying errors and have an eye for detail.

- Logical, analytical and numerical – this often means they are technically very able.

- Honest, with a strict moral code where they tend not cut corners.

- Very motivated by a set routine or method, clear expectation and tend not to get bored by this.

- Keen not to waste time chatting and socialising, instead preferring to get on with the job.

- Happy to work independently.

However, the work situation also presents Daniel with some challenges due to social communication and interaction and sensory challenges inherent in his diagnosis of autism. Below I have made a number of recommendations for a line manager to support some of these difficulties.

- Explain tasks clearly. Try to be clear and specific avoiding the abstract and hypothetical.

- Don't rely on Daniel's ability to interpret facial expression as this is something he may not pick up on.

- Daniel works best if he is dealing with one task at a time. He is likely to be very good at focusing on one task but poor at multitasking or shifting focus.

- Avoid ambiguous language. Try to avoid ambiguous open-ended questions and be aware Daniel may interpret language literally. Check Daniel understands and give regular feedback on his performance.

- Be aware that those on the autism spectrum often present with increased anxiety levels.

**171**

- Be aware that Daniel may not be particularly good at recognising his own stress levels.

- Daniel also presents with sensory difficulties which may require some consideration at work. In particular, he has heightened sensitivity to noise and light.

- Introduce change gradually and prepare Daniel well in advance.

- Be aware that Daniel finds social situations, when he does not have a specified role, draining.

- Daniel is very honest and direct, which can come across as being too blunt. It is unintentional, so try not to take it personally.

- Appointing a work buddy or mentor can be beneficial.

We would be very happy to be contacted about any of the information contained in this letter.

Yours faithfully,
Dr Trevor Powell

# CHAPTER 9

# After diagnosis

## *Reactions, disclosure, stages and advice*

## People's reactions to getting a diagnosis of autism

The majority of people react positively to receiving a diagnosis of autism; it can be a life-changing event, a shift in perspective, an epiphanic moment. It might be the start of a journey as they set out to ask questions and look for answers, to reconcile past experiences through the lens of autism. One man said, 'It was the best news I ever had in my life… I feel like nothing has changed but everything is different. Everything all of a sudden makes sense. The ugly duck is now a swan'. Other people have made similar comments about the life-changing nature of getting a diagnosis:

- 'It was like somebody turning the lights on. Before my diagnosis I was stumbling around in the dark always bumping into the furniture'.

- 'It was like being in court and getting a not guilty verdict'.

- 'I found the key to my life … The diagnosis set me free to be who I really am'.

- 'It was a kind of eureka moment. Finally, I had a name for the thing that made me feel different'.

- 'Diagnosis has unlocked a different version of me – allowing me to reframe my self-identity'.

My colleague Louise Ackers and I carried out a follow-up research study (Powell and Ackers, 2016) of 74 people who had received a diagnosis in the previous 3 months. One of the questions posed in our study was, 'How did getting a diagnosis make you feel?' The group's written responses were divided into six main themes which were as follows:

1 *Relief*: 73% reported being relieved or pleased, stating: 'I was relieved to have it confirmed'; 'relief that it's not caused by my inadequacy'; 'relief not to be labelled a "weirdo"'; 'it was a relief because for years it was put down to anxiety and depression'; 'it was a relief that it wasn't my fault'.

2 *Positive feelings linked to the sense of self*: 'I feel more empowered'; 'makes me feel glad, stronger, independent'; 'I feel validated'; 'I feel more understood'. One person described an almost euphoric experience: 'I was so happy I could not sleep that night. I was "high" for about two weeks ... the only thing I could compare it with was falling in love'.

3 *Mixed feelings*: 'Relieved but daunted... angry and sad that it wasn't picked up earlier'. 'Initially I felt relieved, but at times I see it as confirmation that I am unlikely ever to be normal'. The process of being diagnosed may trigger reflections about past experiences; some participants described being upset or angry that the diagnosis had not been previously recognised. They stated, 'I was upset because I thought back to many instances in my life and how different and better they would have been if I had been diagnosed earlier in life'; '[I am] very sad to think my life would be far better today if I had known earlier'.

4 *Negative feelings*: this occurred particularly among younger people: 'Shocked because I didn't think I had it'; 'angry that if it's 1 in a 100, why does it have to be me? I'm annoyed'; 'It's a bit depressing – confirmation that I will never feel "normal" or will not "get better"'.

5 *No clear feelings*: approximately 10% described having no immediate emotional reaction to the diagnosis, or not being able to describe or label any emotion. Their comments were, 'It has had no effect – I feel no different'; 'I am not bothered'; 'I don't know how I feel about it'; 'I will have to go away and assimilate it – it takes me a while to work through how I feel'. However, for many in this group, getting a diagnosis had more meaning and impact for family members, friends and clinicians, who now had an explanation for the diagnosed person's behaviour.

6 *Diagnostic disappointment*: there is a small group of people who come along hoping for a diagnosis, but leave disappointed when, instead of getting a full diagnosis, they are described as having traits, residual Asperger's or social communication difficulties. One person summarised, 'I was hoping that the assessment would give me clear answers, but it didn't. I'm disappointed and feel that I'm stuck in limbo'.

A dilemma for the clinician is what name or label to give to a person in the 'subclinical threshold group'. The diagnosing clinician must also decide how broadly to interpret the DSM-V medical classification categories when dealing with a condition on a dimensional scale. Personally, the longer I have been carrying out these diagnostic assessments, the more likely I am to give a full diagnosis, even if the person's profile doesn't completely satisfy criteria in all areas. The reason for this is the increasing awareness of 'the female presentation' and the growing realisation that autistic people can have such different profiles. For example, a person might have reasonable non-verbal social and communication skills but severely restricted, repetitive, inflexible behaviours and sensory issues which have a massive impact on all areas of life; hence a diagnosis becomes helpful.

## What effect does getting a diagnosis have on people's lives?

When asked the question, 'What have been the main effects of the assessment on your life?' four main themes emerged.

1  *It provided understanding and explanation:* This was the overwhelming response, expressed by 83% of respondents. Participants reported, 'It puts the pieces together in my mind ... helps because it explains so much ... I reflected on my past'. Many participants made comments indicating that the diagnosis allowed them to understand themselves better: 'It allows me to understand ... the root of the problem'; 'it answered 50 years' worth of questions'. At times, a diagnosis prompted retrospection and reflection: 'When I look back on my life in the light of the diagnosis, things make more sense'; 'I have spent time retracing awkward moments'; 'Now I know why I have struggled with social situations all these years'. Others commented about the positive effect going forward: 'it enabled me to plan and prepare for situations, knowing how I may react', and 'It has helped me understand these feelings and tick off emotions that I've never really understood before such as guilt'.

2  *It made me feel better about myself:* Participants reported that their sense of worth had improved following diagnosis. For some, the diagnosis provided a greater level of self-acceptance: 'In a very real way, the diagnosis has validated my life and made me able to accept that I am not just a failure with a large IQ'. For many participants, the diagnosis helped them to reattribute blame from self to the diagnosis: 'I am more content with myself because I know it's not my fault'; 'I have permission to accept that I find some things hard'; 'Finally I could stop feeling bad about myself'. Interestingly, in many cases, getting a diagnosis prompted people to act with greater confidence and self-compassion: 'It helped me gain confidence in who I am'; 'Having a diagnosis means I don't have to spend my time trying to fix myself'; 'I can tell my nice but naive psychological therapist that there are things about myself that I can't change. My task is then to accept how I am. It's the way my brain is wired'. For some, feeling better about

themselves led to an improvement in mental health: 'Although I still feel like a misfit, I feel better about myself – my mental health has stabilised'.

3 *Tangible gains and support:* Some described the diagnosis as positively 'opening the way' for tangible gains, including study support, financial benefits, autism-related specialist support and autism friendly working practices. 'It helped me get study support at university'; 'It opened the way for tangible gains… benefits'; 'Improved my job prospects … work must now make reasonable allowances', 'I've got an autism awareness card'. However, others pointed out a lack of support: 'I've found little support out there except voluntary groups and people you meet on the internet', 'The therapist in the mental health service didn't seem to know much about it and wasn't very helpful'.

4 *Relationships affected both positively and negatively:* One man commented, 'Work understands me more now'; another said 'My family understands me more now'. One woman commented on how it had improved her marriage: 'My husband said it doesn't change anything, "I love you for who you are, not a label" but now I can explain to him why I can't do certain things or need the volume turned down. It's brought a positive understanding of each other'. However, although the majority of social responses were positive, there were some negative ones too: 'My boyfriend treats me differently now. I'm more aware of being scrutinised'. There was also an awareness of other people's expectations changing: 'It limits the expectations of others; they watch me more closely and assume I'll never be able to do things at work or home that I can do'.

One lady Anna wrote in to say thank you for the assessment, diagnosis and advice:

> I wanted to write and thank you enormously… I am about to start a new job that I chose with reference to your recommendations and, for the first time in my life, feel confident that I will have an occupation that isn't harmful to me. The job is a Lectureship in… at the University of … I will have about 8 contact hours with students a week and the rest of my work will be self-determined in my own private office where I can control the lighting… etc. Although being told that I had Autism was a relief, it was also a shock and I went through a difficult couple of months emotionally. The diagnosis felt like a life sentence and crystallised my feelings of not knowing who I was - if I've been "pretending to be normal" all my life, who am I? If it's Autism, no amount of trying hard will cure it etc. With time, however, things have improved substantially. Implementing lots of sensory techniques has made a huge difference to my mental health and helped to see how much of what I thought was "hysteria", mania, or

anxiety was actually a meltdown. I have become an avid knitter...I carry a muslin bag of coffee beans around with me and a little bottle of frankincense essential oil. I go nowhere without my sunglasses and pink noise. When I am overwhelmed by something I remind myself it's just a meltdown rather than some sort of neurotic attention-seeking behaviour for secondary gain. This makes it easier to forgive myself. Anyway I just wanted to say thank you for a life-changing diagnosis and for giving me the tools to find a healthy job and get the support I need.

## Disclosure

A major issue for everybody who gets a late-in-life diagnosis is disclosure. There are a number of issues here – why, when, who to and how? There is no absolute right or wrong decision here. Some people tell everybody, some tell nobody – to some degree it depends on the personality of the client, whether they are 'open' or 'closed'. In general, it is better to be honest, but there are many factors to consider, and it is a complex personal decision. Kim (2013) provides a note of caution:

> Disclosure is a sticky issue. My first instinct was, "this is great! I have an explanation for my difficulties. I'll tell everybody and they will be as happy as I am". I later realized that disclosure makes people uncomfortable. Many reassure you that it makes no difference and then proceed to treat you differently. Even with the people that are most accepting you notice little shifts in attitude. Remember it's irrevocable, once you share the news you can't unshare it... Generally, I think it best to initially share with those closest to you, your inner circle. Then deciding who to share with in your outer circle is harder and requires some thought – thinking through the consequences.

In considering when to disclose, Wylie (2015) sensibly suggests that it is important to become more self-aware first. This means developing an understanding of the condition, acknowledging personal strengths and weaknesses and being comfortable with the diagnosis before disclosing to others. It might be a good idea to devise a list of traits and behaviours that can be attributed to autism, for example 'I'm easily agitated in crowds or if people frown, I can't tell if they are sad, angry or lonely etc.'. Then it is sensible to examine the advantages and disadvantages of disclosure.

*Possible advantages of disclosure:*

1 It can help to explain to people the reason why some things are more difficult.

2 It can help to avoid misunderstanding – other people realise the autistic person isn't just 'being difficult'.

3 It may enable people to recognise the person's strengths and open up discussion.

4 It allows the person to obtain support at college, provide financial benefits, access treatment for mental health issues or support for physical health.

5 In work, an employer is legally bound to make 'reasonable adjustments' such as changing the environment to accommodate sensory issues.

6 A disclosure might make the person feel safer and more relaxed because they have brought people into their support corner.

7 It reduces the pressure that concealment brings, helping the person to be their real self, more authentic, no longer needing to pretend.

8 It helps to educate others and increases the proportion of people who understand and know about the condition; this will pave the way for other autistic people to have a smoother ride in the future.

9 In a long-term relationship, intimacy may be improved.

10 It might be a last resort, a risk worth taking, when the person can't bear faking it anymore.

Add your own....
*Possible disadvantages of disclosure:*

1 Other people don't always understand.

2 Once you have told one person it can be difficult to control who they will tell.

3 It might alter perceptions about the person, who they are and what they can do, increasing reservations and doubts about the person's abilities.

4 It might create pity or worry that the person is not up to the task in hand.

5 It might increase the risk of being further ostracised, or seen as 'damaged goods', making the person more vulnerable to being discriminated against.

6 It can make the person feel more vulnerable and exposed

7 Some people have no knowledge of autism and hold false stereotypes, leading them to reach faulty conclusions and potentially causing hurt.

Add your own....
Willey (1999) suggests that disclosure has to be dealt with by two groups: those who need to know and those who might not need to know. The need to know group includes those in a position of authority, such as employers, teachers and doctors. Others who need to know are those who provide advice

and support, trustworthy people who look out for your best interests. The group that might not need to know includes tradespersons, people with whom you only have occasional contact, distant relatives, strangers or acquaintances.

In deciding how to disclose, there are at least two options:

- You can make a 'hard' disclosure or full disclosure, using the words *autistic, Asperger's syndrome or autism spectrum disorder*. Questions may follow, so educate yourself and be prepared to provide more information if required. You might be asked: 'I would never guess, what does it mean?' or 'You don't look autistic to me'. It can be a good idea to prepare a short script, or 'disclosure document', explaining that autism is a neurological condition and how the brain being wired differently might impact on communication, social interaction and sensory processing. Perhaps briefly describe your strengths, challenges and personal recommendations for support or adjustment.

Compile a list using the following headings:

- It helps me when people… (e.g. use short sentences/offer me time to respond etc.).

- I have difficulty when people… (e.g. speak too quickly/interrupt me).

- It may be useful for you to know… (e.g. it takes me longer to process verbal input/group situations; with more than four people it is particularly difficult etc.).

Drew (2017), in his book, '*An Adult with an Autism Diagnosis; A guide to the newly diagnosed*' commented: 'I generally keep the first disclosure short. I say, "I'm on the autism spectrum" and follow this up with, "It means I struggle with social situations". And that is all. Later, if they're interested and ask about it, I might start to explain further and later still go into greater depth'.

Soft disclosure is the process of revealing certain difficulties or specific symptoms rather than 'hard disclosure' of a specific diagnosis. One man disclosed to a co-worker about his reluctance to go to a social event: 'I'm good at complex tasks but an idiot at simple things like small talk'. Soft disclosure invites allowances and adjustments by confessing differences but avoids the disability label which can be potentially seen as somewhat stigmatising. A 'drip effect', where information is given gradually, on a need-to-know basis, can also be advantageous. At work it might be best to disclose to a trusted colleague first and see how it goes from there. Derek commented,

> I choose not to fully disclose because of the inevitability of being treated like a "case". Instead I am slowly opening up about my autistic traits without giving them a label so that people can treat me as a person who is overfocused and has quirky ways rather than someone who is autistic.

Willey (1999) suggests keeping it short and simple with people who you will only have brief contact with. She explains that she frequently says things like,

> Would you do me a favour? I have a specific learning difficulty that makes it hard for me to understand jargon and abstract concepts. Could you please explain it in a concrete and simple way so I will be more likely to really understand you? I'm not dense; I just have a problem with language and non-verbal communication.

It is important to be prepared for people's reactions. One possibility is that elderly parents might feel slightly guilty that they didn't pick it up before, or be too set in their ways or conservative in their thinking to embrace the truth warmly. One typical reaction is explained by Steven, aged 40, who commented: 'My dad doesn't think it exists'. Other reactions stem from the fact that autism can present subtly to the casual observer: 'There's nothing wrong; it's just the latest psychobabble, or a way of making excuses for yourself'. With friends and acquaintances, it is important to be discerning because there is a lot of misinformation about autism. One unhelpful scenario is that people might confuse an autism diagnosis with a mental illness. For many, an open disclosure may be beneficial and create a certain freedom, especially to partners in a long-term relationship, but 'The truth may set you free' doesn't necessarily set everybody else free.

Coming out, or disclosing at work, can be part of a long process, and it might be better to speak to others first. In one survey, about a third of people said they fully disclosed at work, another third disclosed to just one or two close colleagues and a third group avoided disclosure completely. As stated earlier, autism is recognised as a 'hidden disability' by law, and the Equality Act (2010) offers some protection in the workplace where employees are legally bound to make 'reasonable adjustments'.

## Stages of processing and progress after diagnosis

There appear to be a number of stages that people go through after getting a diagnosis, but they are not applicable to everyone and they may vary in order. A lot depends on the person's preparedness for getting a diagnosis; some people are very knowledgeable, and the diagnosis is more of a confirmation; others are unprepared and surprised. However, getting a diagnosis is often a turning point, a reaching of a destination. In the next stage of the journey it might be helpful to consider some signposts, a guide to keep moving forward.

*Learning more about autism:* A first stage is to learn about autism and how it affects the person individually. To identify which parts of themselves are autistic and which are camouflaging, trying to compromise and fit in. My client David, with whom I had a number of post-diagnostic counselling sessions, once said to me, 'It's really helpful trying to unravel what is autism and what is my depression'. This is a stage where reading about autism, particularly personal narratives written by autistic people, is helpful – look online and perhaps go to workshops or groups.

*Full realisation and acceptance:* It can take time for a diagnosis to sink in, to achieve acceptance of the autistic self and embrace the condition. An initial tendency towards partial acceptance is common, and at other times there is complete denial. When other people say, 'You don't seem very autistic to me', it can trigger doubt in the mind. One man said, 'It took me a good six to eight months to accept the diagnosis… I would therefore not recommend telling acquaintances until you have accepted it yourself'.

*Reflecting and making sense of the past:* It can be useful to reflect on the past, reappraise situations through the new lens of autism and consider why past events transpired as they did. There are often key incidents in a lifetime of memories to consider in the creation of a new 'sense making narrative', a retelling of a life's story. It helps us to discuss and process. Kim (2013, p43) makes the following comment about 'healing your younger self':

> Growing up undiagnosed is hard. There is a lot of pain with knowing you're different but not knowing why… As I worked back through the more difficult aspects of my childhood, I felt I was somehow mothering my younger self – revisiting each moment looking at it in a new light and telling the younger version of me that it wasn't my fault and that I'd done the best I could… Being able to look back on my childhood and see that my behaviours were a result of my brain chemistry and not a result of 'not being good enough' allowed me to heal some lingering insecurities… It may help to imagine your adult self-sharing your new information with your child self as a way to offer comfort or explanation for unhealed childhood wounds.

*Processing mixed feelings and mourning losses:* Mixed feelings may accompany a diagnosis. As stated, often a primary feeling is relief, but then there might be anger at past injustices leading you to apportion blame to yourself or others for not identifying the conditions earlier. An initial over pessimism – 'I'm faulty, I'm broken, I will never fulfil my dreams' could lead to confusion, 'everything in my life has been chucked upside down – what does it all mean?'. A sense of a loss or change of identity – 'the person I thought I was is gone different' and feelings of anger, disappointment and sadness, need to be acknowledged, aired, discussed and processed.

*Recognising strengths and weaknesses:* It is important for all of us to recognise our strengths, whether they are things we do well, or personal qualities, while at the same time recognising weaknesses and situations that challenge us. To use terminology from the business/management world, it might also be helpful to identify 'threats' and 'opportunities' and to look for situations where strengths are maximised and weaknesses minimised.

*Identify a support team:* We all need support, but this is particularly true in the months and years after getting a diagnosis, as adjustment and changes, emotionally and psychologically are likely – it is a stressful period. The person has to decide, 'Who is going to be helpful, who accepts me, who understands me? The team might include a mixture of family, professional clinicians and therapists, others with autism and like-minded friends and peers.

*Identify coping strategies:* Part of the process of self-reflection is identification of coping strategies. Some might be unhelpful, such as drinking to excess or taking illegal drugs, others might be more obviously helpful like exercise, eating a healthy diet or being in nature.

*Making choices:* There are likely to be' decisions and choices to be made. For example, choosing what type of work best maximises strengths and minimises weaknesses or whether to be involved with certain people and not with others. It is important to construct a comfortable environment and living space. One client decided, 'I needed to move out of that noisy flat, the diagnosis helped me realise that it wasn't just my imagination, but I do have a sensory sensitivity over the noise'.

*Disclosure:* We have dealt with this in the previous section and a summary of a few important points would be: think about it first as once shared it can't be unshared; learn and understand how autism affects you first, prepare a short script to those closest to you first and gradually move outwards. There are two ways to disclose: hard/full disclosure, or soft/partial disclosure.

*Being authentic:* This is the stage where the autistic person embraces their own quirks, flaws and foibles and begins to feel more comfortable in their own skin. It involves deciding how much to allow the expression of the autistic self and how much to compromise, camouflage, to play the game and fit in. Camouflaging might help in the short term but can be harmful in the long term by creating chronic stress and mental health problems. Some people become quite militant and refuse to compromise; others take a more pragmatic approach. It involves finding other autistic people and feeling part of that 'group or 'tribe'. Bulluss and Sesterka (2020) in an interesting article on 'Authenticity and Autism' wrote,

> [Being authentic] is about shredding outdated coping behaviours and refraining from shaping ourselves to fit in with others, and that part of the process may involve saying goodbye to people who do not accept us as we are. This can be a painful process, intense vulnerability and grief may emerge as we unravel our lives, disconnect bonds and weave all that remains back together in colours and patterns that better represent who we really are. But what does that mean for us who are different... we are weaving with different threads. It's not impossible but it presents greater challenges... It takes a great deal of assertiveness and courage... our families may not appreciate or understand us leaving family gatherings early to preserve our cognitive energy, just as colleagues may take offence to us opting to work alone rather than as part of a team. Our camouflaging developed as a survival mechanism, a way of hiding our differences and just blending in,

but now is posing an obstacle to our authentic living. Many people do not react favourably to our authentic autistic selves, but there are also autistic spaces that welcome, honour and appreciate our divergences.

## Advice for thriving after diagnosis

At the end of this book, I would like to give the final word to the people this book is about, namely, the people who have received a diagnosis of autism later in life. I've asked all the clients who have attended the last 15 or so 'Being Me' courses (see Appendix 1), 'What advice would you give to others who might be in the same position and had recently received a diagnosis?' There follows some replies, mixed with comments found from research and the autism literature.

### Gain understanding, self-knowledge and self-reflect

- 'Read about it, especially the personal accounts – educate yourself. But bear in mind people are different. I have found reading helps with self-understanding and self-knowledge and identifying what my needs are. Tony Attwood's book is still incredibly useful'.

- 'Go online – join forums. There is an excellent Facebook page/internet site called "The Curly Haired Project". It is able to put things into words which really help me explain to others. The internet is like a classroom full of research and people's stories'.

- 'I found it helpful to reflect on my life up to the point of diagnosis and how I dealt with things. Everything made more sense. I felt that many things that I had been blaming myself for really weren't my fault. I have decided to give myself a break, stop beating myself up and be kinder to myself'.

- 'I found researching it useful. I reflected on my childhood and wove the research into the experiences of my past and it made much more sense'.

- 'I joined Wrong Planet, an online autism forum, and found the people were very welcoming'.

- 'I joined Autism Berkshire and attended a workshop'.

- 'I attended a post-diagnostic support and education group – Being Me – which was helpful in understanding autism, but also in meeting others with similar issues'.

- 'I'm beginning to understand my own needs better. For example, I need time alone and I've made a rule that I will limit any socialising to a maximum of two hours. My advice is: "Recognise your own needs and assertively try to get them met"'.

- 'I researched online ways that I could change my lifestyle in order to reduce my stress and anxiety and to gain a better understanding of why I felt and behave the way I do. For example, I found out a great deal about aphantasia and alexithymia'.

- 'Go to training seminars'.

- 'Get your partner to read stuff about it as well'.

- 'It is an explanation not a label, don't let it define you'.

- 'The more I read, write or talk about autism the more I feel my sense of self evolving and solidifying'.

- 'The self-knowledge I have gained through the diagnostic process has been life changing and has helped me accept myself. Now I'm beginning to make changes to improve my life'.

## Don't forget your strengths

- 'Remind yourself of your autistic strengths. Think of all the successful famous people who have been autistic – brilliant minds that have changed the world. Write down a list of all your strengths – things you can do that others can't'.

- 'Keep a journal to record insights and transformational experiences or write a blog – I find writing therapeutic and it helps me to piece things together'.

- 'Turn hobbies and special interests – your strengths – into therapeutic activities and career opportunities'.

- 'Celebrate your difference. Autism is a design feature – it's good. We are not broken; we are wonderfully unique thinkers. The world needs us to keep you honest'.

- 'Don't get too caught up in the label – I am still "me" with lots of strengths'.

## Seek support

- 'Wherever you are in your journey, you're not alone. There are other adults out there with the same questions, the same confusion, the same doubts, fears, excitement and Aha! moments'.

- 'Immerse yourself into some kind of autistic community, whether it is a group, an online forum or watching videos of people sharing their experience. Being with people or somebody with the same condition is comforting, knowing you are not alone. I find myself saying, "That's how it is for me"'.

- 'I found a therapist who knew about autism, which was helpful for unpicking and challenging all those unhelpful beliefs I have about being useless, bad and difficult. I feel better about myself as a person now – I'm autistic and okay!'.

- 'Join goal orientated social groups, if you want social contact but struggle with unstructured social situations like dinner parties. Join a group where you might have a common goal, such as cycling or archery'.

- 'I talked to close friends and family about the diagnosis and what it meant for my relationships with them. Support from these people was vital and continues to be so'.

- 'I need support in the form of somebody just giving me the occasional prompt, or reminder of how to think and deal with situations.

- 'I would suggest find a support group. The six-week post-diagnostic group was helpful'.

- 'I've got a friend who has agreed to be my "check out person". I can ring her if I'm unsure about something or confused about what someone has said or done'.

- 'At university, my counsellor put me in touch with a friendship group for people with autism.

- 'It's helpful to find a professional clinician who will be supportive'.

- 'I like the idea of having a mentor, an autistic person, who would be positive and would be a guide for the journey I am now on'.

- 'I've got someone allocated as my "buddy" at work who helps me with work social situations'.

- 'I think something needs to be in place for the partner of the person receiving the diagnosis as this revelation can hit both parties equally hard. My partner was negative and concluded that I was damaged goods. What I could have done with is meeting a positive person who could have calmed my partner and inspired me'.

- 'Analyse your family history to identify the genetic path of autism. Finding out there are relatives who might have had the condition made me somehow feel better and more forgiving of myself'.

- 'Let people know who are closest to you first, give "bits" of information'.

## Self-care – learn to look after yourself and your condition

- 'Since getting the diagnosis I've become gentler and more compassionate with myself. I've allowed myself to stim more, less conscious of censoring myself, I push myself less; cut myself slack where I wouldn't have before. It's not because I see myself as disabled but I see myself as a person in need of care'.

- 'The biggest change is that I've resolved to be kind to myself. I've always been so busy pushing myself, getting things right, I often neglected myself'.

- 'Take time out. If you are in a demanding social situation take a break, take a breather for a few minutes. Take a walk around the block, sit in the garden. Have a safe place you can retreat for a while and relax'.

- 'Make yourself comfortable. I find I just can't think unless I've got comfortable trousers on. So if you want, wear sunglasses, ear plugs, communicate via text rather than speaking. Allow yourself to use things that make life easier'.

- 'Find something that is relaxing – my most effective way is to perform my special interest which is cycling. I can think on a bike. Meditation and mindfulness have been useful also'.

- 'I know I need a quiet, serene, relaxing place to live – somewhere to unwind. I moved out of a flat where there were noisy neighbours and traffic'.

- I am more assertive, standing up for myself, expressing myself, sometimes angrily, and setting the matter straight, when people make annoying comments. I've listed the most annoying comments, which are: 'you don't look autistic', or, 'everybody is a little autistic', or, 'autistic people don't feel empathy', and 'autistic people could be normal if they tried harder'.

## Use practical coping strategies

- 'I carry a card (autism alert card) just in case I find myself in a challenging situation and either have a meltdown or shutdown. I've never had to use it but the fact that it's there is comforting'.

- 'I now know why a structured day makes me feel calmer, so every day I have a plan and a list. I also have taught myself to accept that things don't go according to plan and that is not the end of the world. It's normal!'.

- 'Structure is a (non-negotiable) part of each day. What I wear, eat, do – and how – is all planned out in detail. No unknowns go unturned. Structure is logical and safe. It's like a beacon of light that guides and gives me time and place'.

- 'Have a fast getaway in social situation, such as having my car parked nearby or keeping enough money for a taxi, or even sitting on the end of a table rather than in the middle, is important. Just the knowledge that I can leave a social situation, or escape easily, should I want to, makes the social situation less stressful'.

- Having time out or breathers in social situations helps, even if it's just a walk out into the garden or going to the bathroom, sitting on a bench in the park or sitting in my car for ten minutes closing my eyes and taking a few deep breaths'.

- 'Connect more with nature and its healing powers. Most autistic people are peaceful people who enjoy nature and animals'.

- 'Live in a foreign country or marry a person from a different culture. In Germany many people are 'blunt'. This helps because people from a different culture are less aware and less concerned by our differences'.

- 'My special interests help me stay sane in a world that is baffling and complex. They provide predictability, focus and great reward'.

- 'I shop online and get home delivery, which makes life so much easier'.

- 'I reviewed my employment and took steps to find work that was low stress with an environment that suited my sensory needs'.

- 'I don't communicate with people when I'm angry. I will delay sending that email for 24 hours, and then moderate it'.

- 'I carry a small notebook and Post-it stickers to help with my organisational problems'.

- 'Goal orientated social activities help overcome my social weakness. I struggle where there is no goal other than to socialise, where there are no rules, such as going to a bar or dinner party. I like going to an evening class or my amateur dramatics group or my running club, where there is a shared task and a common topic to discuss'.

- 'It's OK to say you need help. It took me a long time to master this!'.

- 'Prepare stock phrases to take the fear out of conversations and keep the flow such as: "How are you?" Or if there is something I don't understand, I'll sometimes say: "In the sense of..." and trail leaving them to clarify, or I may say: "How do you mean?". If someone asks me how I am and I'm not feeling great I'll say "hanging in there" or "can't complain" or "still breathing"'.

- 'I use humour and gently make fun of my idiosyncrasies before anybody else does'.

- 'I take off my glasses in the supermarket, making the lights and colours much less overwhelming'.

- Do what makes you feel comfortable whatever that might be. It might mean wearing sunglasses indoors, wearing earplugs, sending texts and emails rather than communicating on the phone.

### The way forward towards being more authentic

- 'Everything is a balancing act. I recognise that I have to get a balance between having one foot in the neurotypical world and having one foot in the autistic world and being myself. I don't think that the two extremes of either being an outright autism militant, walking around not compromising or hiding away and feeling bad about yourself are helpful. I would suggest the midpoint, which is to be yourself enough to stay sane, but to compromise with the neurotypical world enough to get by – to be bicultural'.

- 'I initially reflected on the past injustices and problems I'd had through the lens of my new diagnosis, which was painful and made me feel angry and sad. Now I've moved on and am beginning to recognise my strengths, acknowledging which parts of me I accept which parts to change and which parts cannot be changed. I feel I'm moving into new areas of fulfilment'.

- 'Love and accept your own individuality and things will fall into place. Don't deny you have autism as it only makes the world a harder place to live in'.

- 'It's about finding a niche'.

- 'Autistic people are the ultimate square pegs, and the problem with pounding a square into a round hole, is not that the hammering is hard work. It's that you destroy the peg'.

- 'My way forward is about being the most authentic version of yourself that I can be. The largest part of the journey has been accepting myself the way I am and to stop desperately trying to fit in. I am who I am, I'm autistic and proud. I'm different, but that's okay'.

- 'Don't expect everybody to understand and believe you. Be aware that people don't understand autism, even professionals'.

- 'You've always been autistic and you always will be. But that doesn't mean you can't work on learning social skills and emotional intelligence, developing coping mechanisms or change your lifestyle/environment in ways that support you'.

- 'Beware of the peaks and troughs of mood. Sometimes I think I am getting somewhere and then feel that I'm at the bottom of the learning curve again'.

- 'I decided to be a first-rate Aspie rather than a second rate nuero-typical'.

- 'It took me a time to emotionally process it, but then I realised, "I'm different not defective, stop beating yourself up", that was a big mental and emotional shift. Not only am I different but I've gradually met other people similar to me. It's taken me years, but I've gradually become more comfortable in my own skin'.

- 'On any given day, I can be just like everyone else seems to be. Until I remember that I do not have to be. The me that I am has finally made friends with the differences I no longer try to hide' (Willey, 1999, p112).

# Appendix 1

## 'Being Me' group: Exercises for a 6-week post-diagnostic course

This section consists of a number of handouts which form the basis of a 6-week post-diagnostic course, 'Being Me'. The exercises can be used either by a group or by an individual. If working as an individual, you might like to seek the support of your partner, relative or friend. The exercises and group and individual processes are aimed at helping people in the following areas:

1 Develop self-awareness, self-reflection and process the diagnosis.

2 Structure a pathway to move forward.

3 Meet others in a similar position and identify similar experiences.

4 Learn and understand more about autism.

5 Learn and share coping strategies with others.

Each session usually lasts for 2 hours with a short break in the middle. The ideal number in a group ranges from six to nine. Each session would normally have two or three items and handouts for discussion and to work through. Most people are very anxious to start off with but by the end of the course are more relaxed, exchanging telephone numbers and email addresses. Our experience is that people like structure in the group and the emphasis on practical suggestions for help.

Week 1: autism awareness – reaction to getting a diagnosis

Week 2: how does autism affect me – sensory sensitivities – positive aspects

Week 3: disclosure – socialising – special interests

Week 4: employment – getting a balance

Week 5: understanding your emotions – empathic attunement – communication

Week 6: being less rule-bound – reappraising negative messages – advice going forward

# Autism quiz and definitions

*Exercise 1:* Autism quiz. Read each statement in the following section and state whether it is true or false. *Discuss/consider.*

| Autism is ... | True | False |
| --- | :---: | :---: |
| 1  caused by stress | ☐ | ☐ |
| 2  associated with different wiring/connectivity in the brain | ☐ | ☐ |
| 3  more common in boys than girls | ☐ | ☐ |
| 4  the result of unaffectionate parents | ☐ | ☐ |
| 5  often associated with repetitive behaviour | ☐ | ☐ |
| 6  a condition that is prevalent in just over 1% of the population | ☐ | ☐ |
| 7  six times more likely to occur if the father is over 40 | ☐ | ☐ |
| 8  sometimes associated with genius | ☐ | ☐ |
| 9  something you are born with | ☐ | ☐ |
| 10 a mental health issue | ☐ | ☐ |

Answers on the final page of the book.

*Exercise 2:* Which definition do you prefer? Read each definition and rank in order which you like best to worst. *Consider/discuss.*

(a) Autism involves differences/difficulties in social communication and usually strong, narrow interests, repetitive behaviour and sensory sensitivities.

(b) 'Autism' comes from the Greek word *'autos'*, meaning 'self'. The condition implies a lack of understanding of others – or difficulty 'putting yourself in somebody else's shoes', or seeing the world from the perspective of another.

(c) 'The autistic brain is highly wired in the areas involved with attention to detail, memory and systematizing – like an eight-lane motorway. But, in areas concerned with the social and emotional world, the connections are less densely wired – rather like a country lane'.

## Being on the autism spectrum: Language and labels

Somebody once said, 'If you haven't got a word for it, it doesn't exist'. One of the issues with autism is which words or diagnostic labels to use.

*Exercise 1:* Which names or diagnostic labels do you prefer when referring to yourself? *Consider/discuss.*

Rank on a 5-point scale:
1 = strongly dislike; 2 = dislike; 3 = neither like nor dislike; 4 = like; 5 = strongly like.

| | | | |
|---|---|---|---|
| Autistic person | ☐ | Person with autism | ☐ |
| On the autistic spectrum | ☐ | Asperger's syndrome | ☐ |
| Autistic spectrum disorder | ☐ | Autistic spectrum condition | ☐ |
| Aspie | ☐ | ASD | ☐ |

*Exercise 2:* What factors led to you seeking a diagnosis?

_____

_____

_____

_____

*Exercise 3:* How would you describe your 'being on the spectrum' to somebody else if asked?

_____

_____

_____

_____

*Exercise 4:* What would you like to learn about being on the autism spectrum?

_____

_____

_____

_____

# Feelings about getting a diagnosis

The majority of people who seek a diagnosis later in life have mixed feelings but often feel a sense of relief on getting the diagnosis.

*Exercise 1:* How did you feel about getting a diagnosis? (Tick the relevant boxes)

| 1 Relieved | ☐ | 5 Confused | ☐ | 9 Depressed | ☐ |
|---|---|---|---|---|---|
| 2 Angry | ☐ | 6 Shocked | ☐ | 10 Upset | ☐ |
| 3 Elated | ☐ | 7 Anxious | ☐ | 11 Alone | ☐ |
| 4 Nothing | ☐ | 8 Frustrated | ☐ | 12 Surprised | ☐ |

Please list any other feelings you had.

_____

_____

_____

*Exercise 2:* Write a sentence that best describes your emotional reaction to getting a diagnosis.

_____

_____

_____

*Exercise 3:* What aspect of your life has been most positively affected by getting a diagnosis? What have been the negative aspects?

_____

_____

_____

*Exercise 4:* Do you agree with this statement? *Consider/discuss.*
'People with autism are just different, not disabled. We don't want a cure, treatment or sympathy, just acceptance'.

_____

_____

_____

# How does being on the autism spectrum affect me?

Every autistic person is different. It is important to understand your own profile of strengths and challenges.

---

*Exercise 1:* Read the following statements and tick the boxes next to the statements that best describe you – tick as many boxes as appropriate. *Consider/discuss.*

---

1  I have special focussed interests that I can be very passionate about. ☐

2  I am very honest, which has at times got me into trouble, without ☐ meaning to.

3  I find it difficult to tell if someone listening to me is getting bored. ☐

4  When I read a story I find it difficult to work out the characters' ☐ intentions.

5  I prefer sameness and consistency and my predictable routine. ☐

6  I enjoy my own company and often find social situations challenging. ☐

7  I find it hard to tell when other people are joking or being sarcastic. ☐

8  I prefer interesting conversations rather than random 'chit chat' or ☐ 'small talk'.

9  I am very sensitive to touch or certain textures or smells or ☐ particular noises.

10  I often find it hard to know what other people are feeling and ☐ thinking.

11  I usually concentrate more on the details rather the whole picture. ☐

12  If there is an interruption, I find it difficult to switch back to what I ☐ was doing.

13  I find it difficult to 'read between the lines' when someone is ☐ talking to me.

14  I have a very sensitive palate resulting in very specific food ☐ preferences.

---

*Exercise 2:* Add one more statement about yourself – either a strength or challenge.

---
---
---
---
---

## Sensory sensitivities

*Exercise:* Fill out the table to work out what your sensory sensitivities are (if you have any) and how you could cope with them. *Consider/discuss.*

| Sense | Sensitivity | Coping strategy |
|---|---|---|
| | *(e.g. 'I don't like rough fabric on my skin')* | *(e.g. 'I cut out labels in clothes and avoid wool')* |
| **Sounds** | | |
| **Taste** | | |
| **Touch** | | |
| **Vision** | | |
| **Smell** | | |
| **Coordination and balance** | | |
| **Temperature** | | |
| **Pain** | | |
| **Any other** | | |

# Positive aspects of being on the autism spectrum

Some autistic people have a wide range of heightened abilities which sometimes gives an advantage in certain areas of life and work. Think about feedback given by others.

*Exercise 1:* Tick any of the boxes next to the sentences below that describe you best.

**Focus**
- ☐ I am good at noticing details.
- ☐ I can concentrate intensely for long periods.

**Memory**
- ☐ I have good long-term memory.
- ☐ I have a good memory for facts or figures.

**Accepting of difference**
- ☐ I am non-judgemental and accept others.

**Expertise**
- ☐ I know a lot about my hobby or interest.

**Integrity**
- ☐ I'm very honest and don't lie.

**Creativity**
- ☐ I have a distinctive imagination.
- ☐ I have unique thought processes.

**Methodical approach**
- ☐ I am good at following rules.
- ☐ I am a bit of a 'perfectionist' – I like to get things right.
- ☐ I like to get on with the job/finish a task.

Every experience of autism is unique. No one person will identify with every positive feature of autism.

*Exercise 2:* Describe something you are particularly good at or a special skill or interest you have that is in some way linked to your autism.

_____

_____

_____

*Exercise 3:* Discuss/consider the names and achievements of other autistic people who have been successful. *For example, Albert Einstein and his theory of relativity and Susan Boyle singer.*

_____

_____

## Disclosure

There are no hard-and-fast rules about disclosure, but bear in mind the following:

- Consider carefully who to tell – it is irrevocable, once shared you can't unshared.

- Learn about autism and yourself first, so you can respond to questions.

- Share with those closest (inner circle) before considering others (outer circle).

- Decide whether to give a full (hard) disclosure or a partial (soft) disclosure.

- Have someone to discuss issues with and offer support.

Look at section in Chapter 9 on advantages and disadvantages of disclosure  page 177 and consider/discuss the advantages and disadvantages of disclosure

---

*Exercise 1:* Identify people in your inner and outer circle.

Who would you tell and why?

Who have you already told? What was their reaction?

*Consider/discuss.*

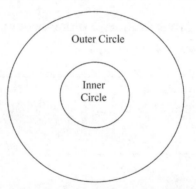

---

*Exercise 2:* 'Soft disclosure' is how to disclose information without using a full label. A person with poor eye contact could say, 'The reason I'm not looking at you is because I have a sensory integration disorder and find it difficult to look and listen at the same time. I am listening to every word that you say'.

Prepare a sentence of what you might say to people you disclose to as an example of 'soft disclosure'.

_____

_____

_____

_____

## Socialising

---

*Exercise 1:* Which social skills do you find challenging and need to work on improving?

| Social skill | Yes | No |
|---|---|---|
| 1  Using eye contact | ☐ | ☐ |
| 2  How to start a conversation | ☐ | ☐ |
| 3  Talking about my interests with passion, for too long | ☐ | ☐ |
| 4  Where to stand when talking to people | ☐ | ☐ |
| 5  How to show people you're listening to them | ☐ | ☐ |
| 6  Knowing when you should/shouldn't interrupt | ☐ | ☐ |
| 7  Not changing the subject too much when talking | ☐ | ☐ |
| 8  Being very honest, sometimes too honest | ☐ | ☐ |
| 9  How to recognise what might upset people | ☐ | ☐ |
| 10  How to end a conversation | ☐ | ☐ |
| 11  Struggling with chit-chat, preferring interesting conversation | ☐ | ☐ |

---

*Exercise 2:* One way to successfully start a conversation is to think, 'what do people talk about?' (WORM). Give an example for something to talk about for each topic.

**W**eather _____

**O**ccupation _____

**R**ecreation _____

**M**edia _____

---

*Exercise 3:* What are the difficulties with small talk? Consider/discuss how you cope. (E.g. *I have a prepared script...* or *I deliberately note something interesting from the newspaper or social media to talk about.*)

_____

_____

_____

## Special focussed interests

Many people on the autism spectrum have special, focussed, passionate interests and expertise that bring a great deal of pleasure and relaxation.

*Exercise 1:* For this exercise, find people to work with. Each should list five interests as shown in the table and then discuss them together and with the group.

| Person A | Person B |
|----------|----------|
| 1 | 1 |
| 2 | 2 |
| 3 | 3 |
| 4 | 4 |
| 5 | 5 |

*Exercise 2:* Write down three main reasons why interests can be useful (e.g. in times of stress they help me relax and distract me from the stress).

1 _____

2 _____

3 _____

_____

*Exercise 3:* Can you think of any special intense interests you had when you were younger that you may have moved on from or still have?

_____

_____

_____

_____

## Employment

*Exercise 1:* Identify areas of work where you need support – try to make specific suggestions about possible 'reasonable adjustments' management at work could make.

| **Area where I need support** (e.g. working in open plan office too distracting) | **Reasonable adjustments** (e.g. allowed seat by window and to wear headphones) |
|---|---|
| _____ | _____ |
| _____ | _____ |
| _____ | _____ |

*Exercise 2:* Identify a problem that has occurred at work before getting your diagnosis and then try to describe in hindsight how you could cope with it better since your diagnosis.

| **Problem** | **How would you cope now** |
|---|---|
| _____ | _____ |
| _____ | _____ |
| _____ | _____ |

*Exercise 3:* List your strengths in the first column. Then, think about possible jobs that may be relevant to those interests. Maximise your strengths/interests, minimise your weaknesses.

| **Interests/strengths** | **Possible job** |
|---|---|
| _____ | _____ |
| _____ | _____ |
| _____ | _____ |

# Energy bank account – getting a balance

Energy levels are like a bank account. Some activities withdraw and drain, leaving you fatigued, while some activities are like a deposit – they add to and refresh your account.

*Exercise 1:* Consider and identify activities that withdraw energy and those that deposit energy.

| *Examples of withdrawers/drainers* | | *Examples of deposits/refreshers* | |
|---|---|---|---|
| Socialising | Sensory sensitivities | Special interests | Sleep |
| Crowds | Being anxious | Physical activity | Caring for others |
| Certain people | Changes | Solitude | Computer games |
| Making a mistake | Being teased | Being in nature | Certain people |
| People's moods | Perceived injustices | Being with a pet | Surfing Internet |
| Add… | | Add… | |

*Exercise 2:* Plan your account, to balance 'drainers' with 'refreshers' for a day.

| *Withdrawers/drainers* | *Deposits/refreshers* |
|---|---|
| E.g. team meeting at lunch time | E.g. walking the dog for 40 minutes |
| • | • |
| • | • |
| • | • |
| • | • |
| • | • |

# Understanding your emotions

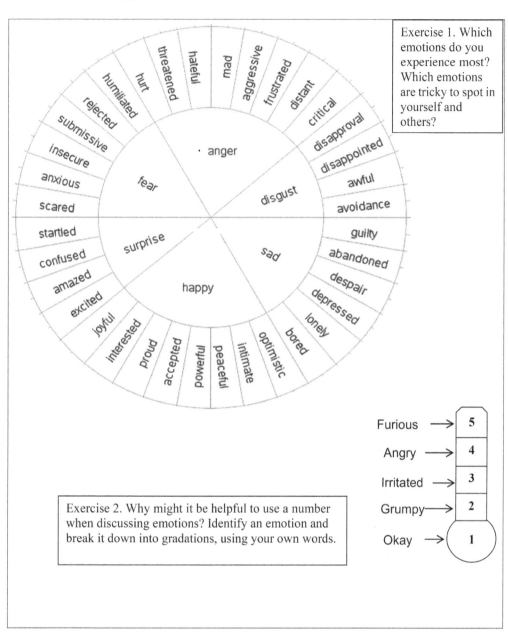

Exercise 1. Which emotions do you experience most? Which emotions are tricky to spot in yourself and others?

Exercise 2. Why might it be helpful to use a number when discussing emotions? Identify an emotion and break it down into gradations, using your own words.

Furious → 5
Angry → 4
Irritated → 3
Grumpy → 2
Okay → 1

# Empathic attunement

Empathy or 'emotional intelligence' is our ability to identify what someone is thinking and feeling and to respond. It has three components: thinking, feeling and behaviour.

---

*Exercise 1:* Rate your own empathy. Circle the option that best applies to you.

| | | | |
|---|---|---|---|
| Thinking: recognising cues for distress in others | Good | Average | Poor |
| Feeling: feeling emotions for others | Good | Average | Poor |
| Behaviour: acting compassionately | Good | Average | Poor |

---

*Exercise 2:* Here are some strategies, others have suggested, for improving empathic attunement or 'emotional intelligence'. Which statements do you identify with most, if any? *Consider/discuss.*

1 I say to myself, 'What would another person feel or do in this situation?'

2 I might admit to the person, 'I'm here because I care, but I don't know what to do to help'.

3 I have specifically learned about emotions, what they feel like and what situations they occur in.

4 I remind myself to try to think how the other person is feeling, not just myself.

5 I have learned by copying others, watching TV and films and have learned to say things like 'Oh dear' and 'Mmm'.

6 I try to be practically helpful, e.g. make a cup of tea.

7 I have found a therapist who is helping with my emotional understanding.

8 Add any others.

---

*Exercise 3:* Claire said, 'I don't always notice other people's moods, but sometimes when I do I get completely overwhelmed with compassion and empathy for the other person. Sometimes my processing of emotions is delayed and sometimes it feels as if I catch people's anger or sadness almost as if it's contagious, like catching a cold'. *Consider/discuss.*

---

# Communication

*Exercise 1:* In general communication, what information might you miss or misunderstand? Tick those that apply:

- The story line of books and films ☐
- Picking up on sarcasm ☐

- Interpreting tone of voice ☐
- A look or facial expressions ☐

- *Add others*

---

*Exercise 2:* What strategies might be helpful in these situations of communication breakdown?

- In an emotional argument to text or write down my thoughts and feelings.
- In a meeting at work to ask for an agenda in advance.
- To get a trusted colleague to check certain emails before I send them.
- *Add others*

---

*Exercise 3:* Communication breaks down frequently for everyone. In what situations is communication likely to break down for you? Tick those situations that apply:

- When I get bored and am not interested. ☐
- When I don't know what to say. ☐
- When sensory difficulties get in the way (e.g. noise). ☐
- When I get anxious/stressed. ☐
- *Add others*

---

*Exercise 4:* The term 'rescue phrases' are comments that acknowledge communication difficulties and allow the person you are communicating with to understand what is specifically challenging – e.g.:

- Sorry, could you say that again? I am not sure I've understood.
- Can I just clarify what you said, so I understand?
- Can you give me a moment to think about that?
- *Add others*

---

## Being less rule-bound

*Exercise 1:* **Annie's dilemma:** When I'm at work I am always very punctual and never like being late. However, although this can be viewed as a positive attribute there is also a flip side to it. If somebody was late for a meeting I'd think that it was rude and disrespectful. I'd find it very difficult to get over my anger, which often spoils the event and my contribution.

How would you advise Annie in trying to overcome the problem of getting stressed? What could she do to 'let it go' – what thoughts could she challenge, or how could she behave differently?

_____

_____

_____

_____

_____

*Exercise 2:* Which of these strategies to loosen up your behaviour can you identify with?

- I try to distract myself by doing something different.

- I breathe slowly and make a conscious decision to stop my mind racing.

- I try to ignore it and make excuses for others.

- I try to replace the word 'they should' with 'it would be nice if…'.

- I tell the person it really upsets me.

- I say to myself, 'people are different' and try to accept it.

- I ask myself what somebody else (e.g. Mr Spock from *Star Trek*) would think and do.

- I try to make a joke (e.g. saying, 'I'm a control freak').

- I say the Serenity Prayer to myself, realising I can't do anything about it.

- (God, grant me the serenity to accept the things I cannot change, courage to change the things I can, and wisdom to know the difference).

- Add your own strategies. *Consider/discuss.*

# Reappraising negative messages

A period of thinking about the past often accompanies a diagnosis. This might include remembering hurtful criticism. For example, being told that you are 'difficult' or 'awkward' after behaving in a particular way. Those judgemental, shaming messages could be reappraised in the light of a diagnosis of autism and rewritten as, 'No, I'm not difficult, I acted as I did because I am autistic': strike out the word 'difficult' and replace it with 'autistic'. Discuss the following examples:

- 'I struggle with the concept of time because ~~I lack boundaries~~ I am autistic'.

- 'I sometimes don't pick up on people's moods because ~~I am selfish~~ I am autistic'.

- 'I need to have the details of plans because ~~I am difficult~~ I am autistic'.

- 'I frequently interrupt during meetings because ~~I am rude~~ I am autistic'.

---

*Exercise 1:* Identify thoughts you have about yourself (as earlier) based on the negative comments of others, e.g. I... (do something) because I am ~~'difficult'~~, ~~'awkward'~~ etc. and change the negative word to 'autistic'.

- 

- 

- 

---

*Exercise 2:* Think of a situation from the past where you struggled or didn't cope and then blamed yourself and felt bad. Rewrite or reappraise that situation, explaining the reasons for your difficulties in terms of your autism.

_____

_____

_____

_____

# Advice for somebody who has just received a diagnosis of autism

*Exercise 1:* What advice would you give to someone who has just received a diagnosis of autism? Read the suggestions and rate how helpful you think these suggestions would be
(3 = very helpful; 2 = helpful; 1 = not helpful).

1  Read as much as possible about it – also include your partner.  ☐
2  Join a post-diagnostic support group/support network.  ☐
3  Expect emotional ups and downs.  ☐
4  Join an Internet site or forum.  ☐
5  Keep a journal or diary, noting changes and making connections.  ☐
6  Carry an 'autism alert' card, just in case.  ☐
7  Try to spend time with supportive professionals or clinicians.  ☐
8  Be careful about disclosure.  ☐
9  Attend training workshops and conferences on autism.  ☐
10 Be aware that some people, even professionals, don't understand autism.  ☐
11 It's an explanation, not a label. Don't let it define you.  ☐
12 Strive to be your authentic autistic self – compromise, but not excessively.  ☐

*Exercise 2:* What advice would you give to somebody who has just had a diagnosis and what have you found helpful? *Consider/discuss.*

_____

_____
_____

_____

*Exercise 3:* Do you recognise any emotional stages or processes that you have been through since getting your diagnosis? *Consider/discuss.*

_____

_____
_____

*Exercise 4:* The way forward. Identify two personal goals for the next year, which are specific tasks and which goals you will use to attempt to improve the quality of your life following your diagnosis.

_____

_____
_____

# Appendix 2

## *Glossary*

Understanding medical and technical terms

**Alexithymia**   a condition where an individual struggles to find words for their emotions

**Amygdala**   a part of the brain associated with emotions

**Asperger's syndrome**   a different name for people with autism, without a learning difficulty

**Aspie**   a colloquial term for someone who has Asperger's syndrome

**Attention deficit hyperactivity disorder (ADHD)**   a set of behavioural symptoms that include difficulties with attention, hyperactivity and impulsiveness

**Autistic spectrum disorder (ASD)**   a term used to describe all the variations of autism. A condition characterised by difficulties with social interaction, communication and behaviour.

**Bipolar disorder**   a mental health condition, characterised by alternating periods of mania and depression

**Borderline personality disorder (BPD)**   a type of personality characterised by difficulty forming and keeping stable relationships, impulsivity and shifting moods

**Camouflaging**   disguise, mask, make blend in with surroundings

**Cerebellum**   a part of the brain located at the back of the head involved in the control of movement, balance, motor coordination and social cognition

**Clinical psychologist**   the branch of psychology dealing with diagnosis and treatment of mental health conditions

**Cognition**   the mental process of thought based on knowledge and understanding

**Cognitive behavioural therapy (CBT)**   a common therapy to treat conditions like anxiety and depression that aims to help one to teach people how to manage emotions by changing the way they think and feel

**Co-morbidities** mental health conditions that co-occur or occur simultaneously

**DSM-V** *The Diagnostic and Statistical Manual of Mental Disorders:* 5th Edition. American dictionary of diagnosis

**Dyscalculia** difficulty understanding even basic mathematical concepts

**Dyslexia** a specific learning difficulty affecting the ability to read and spell

**Dyspraxia** a developmental condition characterised by difficulty involving coordination, movement, planning and organising

**Echolalia** repetition of speech or words

**Empathy** understanding and sharing feelings of another

**Epilepsy** a neurological condition associated with abnormal electrical activities in the brain resulting in episodes of sensory disturbance and loss of consciousness

**Executive functioning** skills located in the frontal lobes of the brain involved in planning and organising, multitasking and problem solving

**Frontal lobes** area of brain behind forehead concerned with behaviour, personality, thinking and executive skills

**Fusiform gyrus** area in the temporal lobe, thought to be important in facial recognition and facial expression

**Gender dysphoria** distress that accompanies incongruence between experienced gender and birth sex

**Hyperlexia** an advanced ability at reading and recognising words, without prior training and comprehension of the words – a 'superability'

**Hypersensitive** oversensitive

**Hyposensitive** undersensitive

**ICD-10** *The International Statistical Classification of Diseases and Related Health Problems:* 10th Edition

**Incidence** the actual number of people with a confirmed diagnosis

**Insula** area of the brain that receives signals from organs of the body and forms a map of sensation

**Intermediary** professional who facilitates communication between the police, judiciary and witness

**Interoception** the ability to detect and attend to bodily sensations

**Learning disability (LD)** a condition associated with learning difficulties, reduced intellectual ability and difficulty with everyday activities

**Meltdown** an uncontrolled emotional outburst or collapse

**Monotropism** theory suggesting autism is essentially about paying attention to what is in his or her attention tunnel

**Neurodevelopmental** relating to the development of the nervous system

**Neurotypical** a term used to describe non-autistic people and their thinking style

**Obsessive compulsive disorder (OCD)** an anxiety disorder associated with obsessions and compulsions

**Olfactory** sense of smell

**Pedantic speech** overly formal speech

**Personality disorder** a condition associated with difficulties with relationships and functioning in society

**Pragmatic aspects of language** the modification and use of language in a social context

**Prevalence** the number of people in the general population who have the condition

**Proprioception** the unconscious perception of movement and spatial orientation of the body, limbs and head

**Prosody** the vocal tone and quality of speech

**Prosopagnosia** face blindness

**Psychiatrist** a medical practitioner specialising in the diagnosis and treatment of mental health conditions

**Psychosis** a mental health condition associated with symptoms such as delusions or hallucinations that suggest impaired contact with reality

**Purkinje cells** nerve cells, found in the cerebellum, involved with motor coordination

**Savant skills** exceptional ability generally related to memory

**Schizophrenia** mental health condition characterised by withdrawal from reality, illogical patterns of thinking, delusions, behaviours and psychotic behaviour

**Sensory sensitivities** sensitivity with processing sensory information, such as sound, sight, smell, taste and touch

**Stimming** self-stimulating behaviour (flapping hands, licking, spinning, rocking) designed to calm or de-stress

**Synaesthesia** a rare form of sensory perception where two or more sensory experiences are linked (e.g. colour–number)

**Systematising** the drive to analyse or build a system that follows rules

**Temporal lobe** an area of the brain involved with among other things sound perception, speech, language and memory

**Theory of mind (ToM)** the ability to recognise and understand other people's thoughts, feelings and intentions to understand their behaviour

**Tics** occasional, involuntary movements or sounds

**Tourette's syndrome** a neurological condition, characterised by involuntary tics and vocalisations

**Weak central coherence** difficulty understanding the overall picture of something and instead focusing on parts

# Appendix 3
## Useful contacts, organisations and websites

Tony Attwood's website: www.tonyattwood.com.au

*National Autistic Society:* This national organisation provides support, information and services to individuals with ASD, their families and professionals: www.autism.org.uk Tel: +44 (0) 20 7833 2299. Helpline: 08450 704 004

*Autistica*: London-based autism charity: www.autistica.org.uk

*Autism Research Centre (ARC):* https://www.autismresearchcentre.com/. The mission of ARC is to understand the causes of autism and develop new methods for assessment and intervention.

*The Curly Hair Project:* Aims to help women and girls and their neurotypical loved ones communicate and understand each other better: https://thegirlwiththecurlyhair.co.uk/

*Scottish Autism online program:* Free resource for women, girls, parents and carers: http://www.scottishautism.org/services-support/support-families/women-and-girls-online-support

Armstrong (2011) The Power of Neurodiversity: Unleashing the Advantages of Your Differently Wired Brain
https://www.youtube.com/watch?v=aWxmEv7fOFY
https://www.youtube.com/watch?v=Qvvrme5WIwA

University of Exeter research project called Exploring Diagnosis: Autism and Neurodiversity have made three short films: https://www.youtube.com/results?search_query=%23ExDxFilms.

*Jessica Kingsley Publishers:* Leading publisher for autism books: www.jkp.com

*Sensory Processing Foundation:* USA website with information about Sensory processing, tips and research: http://spdfoundation.net/

Wrong Planet a web community designed for individuals (as well as their families and professionals) with AS and other neurological difficulties: Website: www.wrongplanet.net

Good for sensory processing – young person: https://eatingoffplastic.wordpress.com/

# Appendix 4

## The adult autism-spectrum quotient (AQ)

Reproduced with kind permission from the Autism Research Unit University of Cambridge. For full details, see Baron-Cohen S, Wheelwright S, Skinner R, Martin J & Clubley E (2001) 'The autism spectrum quotient (AQ): evidence from Asperger syndrome/high functioning autism, males and females, scientists and mathematicians', *Journal of Autism and Developmental Disorders*, 31, pp5–17. This is downloadable from http://autismresearchcentre.com. This is a screening and research tool, not a direct diagnostic tool.

The AQ is provided for research use only and should not be used to inform clinical decisions. Any commercial use of the AQ is prohibited without prior express written permission from the creators and the Autism Research Centre at the University of Cambridge.

*Responses that score 1 point are marked. Other responses score 0. For total score, sum all item*

| | | Definitely agree | Slightly agree | Slightly disagree | Definitely disagree |
|---|---|---|---|---|---|
| 1 | I prefer to do things with others rather than on my own | | | 1 | 1 |
| 2 | I prefer to do things the same way over and over again | 1 | 1 | | |
| 3 | If I try to imagine something, I find it easy to create a picture in my mind | | | 1 | 1 |
| 4 | I frequently get so strongly absorbed in one thing that I lose sight of other things | 1 | 1 | | |
| 5 | I often notice small sounds when others do not | 1 | 1 | | |
| 6 | I usually notice car number plates or similar things of information | 1 | 1 | | |
| 7 | Other people frequently tell me that what I've said is impolite, even though I think it is polite | 1 | 1 | | |

| | | Definitely agree | Slightly agree | Slightly disagree | Definitely disagree |
|---|---|---|---|---|---|
| 8 | When I'm reading a story, I can easily imagine what the characters might look like | | | 1 | 1 |
| 9 | I am fascinated by dates | 1 | 1 | | |
| 10 | In a social group, I can easily keep track of several different people's conversations | | | 1 | 1 |
| 11 | I find social situations easy | | | 1 | 1 |
| 12 | I tend to notice details that others do not | 1 | 1 | | |
| 13 | I would rather go to a library than go to a party | 1 | 1 | | |
| 14 | I find making up stories easy | | | 1 | 1 |
| 15 | I find myself drawn more strongly to people than things | | | 1 | 1 |
| 16 | I tend to have very strong interests, which I get upset about if I can't pursue | 1 | 1 | | |
| 17 | I enjoy social chit-chat | | | 1 | 1 |
| 18 | When I talk, it isn't always easy for others to get a word in edgeways | 1 | 1 | | |
| 19 | I am fascinated by numbers | 1 | 1 | | |
| 20 | When I'm reading a story, I find it difficult to work out the characters' intentions | 1 | 1 | | |
| 21 | I don't particularly enjoy reading fiction | 1 | 1 | | |
| 22 | I find it hard to make new friends | 1 | 1 | | |
| 23 | I notice patterns in things all the time | 1 | 1 | | |
| 24 | I would rather go to the theatre than to a museum | | | 1 | 1 |
| 25 | It does not upset me if my daily routine is disturbed | | | 1 | 1 |
| 26 | I frequently find that I don't know how to keep a conversation going | 1 | 1 | | |
| 27 | I find it easy to 'read between the lines' when someone is talking to me | | | 1 | 1 |
| 28 | I usually concentrate more on the whole picture, rather than on the small details | | | 1 | 1 |
| 29 | I am not very good at remembering phone numbers | | | 1 | 1 |
| 30 | I don't usually notice small changes in a situation, or a person's appearance | | | 1 | 1 |
| 31 | I know how to tell if someone listening to me is getting bored | | | 1 | 1 |
| 32 | I find it easy to do more than one thing at once | | | 1 | 1 |
| 33 | When I talk on the phone, I'm not sure when it's my turn to speak | 1 | 1 | | |
| 34 | I enjoy doing things spontaneously | | | 1 | 1 |
| 35 | I am often the last to understand the point of a joke | 1 | 1 | | |

| | | Definitely agree | Slightly agree | Slightly disagree | Definitely disagree |
|---|---|---|---|---|---|
| 36 | I find it easy to work out what someone is thinking or feeling just by looking at their face | | | 1 | 1 |
| 37 | If there is an interruption, I can switch to what I was doing very quickly | | | 1 | 1 |
| 38 | I am good at social chit-chat | | | 1 | 1 |
| 39 | People often tell me that I keep going on and on about the same thing | 1 | 1 | | |
| 40 | When I was young, I used to enjoy playing games involving pretending with other children | | | 1 | 1 |
| 41 | I like to collect information about categories of things (e.g. types of cars, birds, trains, plants) | 1 | 1 | | |
| 42 | I find it difficult to imagine what it would be like to be someone else | 1 | 1 | | |
| 43 | I like to carefully plan any activities I participate in | 1 | 1 | | |
| 44 | I enjoy social occasions | | | 1 | 1 |
| 45 | I find it difficult to work out people's intentions | 1 | 1 | | |
| 46 | New situations make me anxious | 1 | 1 | | |
| 47 | I enjoy meeting new people | | | 1 | 1 |
| 48 | I am a good diplomat | | | 1 | 1 |
| 49 | I am not very good at remembering people's date of birth | | | 1 | 1 |
| 50 | I find it very easy to play games with children that involve pretending | | | 1 | 1 |

How to interpret your score?

- 0–10 = Low

- 11–22 = Average (most women score around 15 and men score about 17)

- 23–31 = Above average

- 32–50 = Very high (most people with autism score about 35)

- 50 = Maximum

Answers to the autism quiz on page 192: true: 2, 3, 5, 6, 7, 8, 9; false: 1, 4, 10

# Appendix 5
## References

Andrews D (2006) 'Mental health issues surrounding diagnosis and disclosure', Murray D (ed), *Coming Out Asperger: Diagnosis, Disclosure and Self-Confidence*, Jessica Kingsley Publishers, London.

American Psychiatric Association (2013) *The Diagnostic and Statistical Manual of Mental Disorders*: 5th Edition: Washington, DC: *APA*

Asperger H (1944) 'Autistic psychopathy in childhood', Frith U (ed), *Autism and Asperger Syndrome*, Cambridge University Press, Cambridge.

Aston M (2009) *The Asperger Couples Workbook*, Jessica Kingsley Publishers, London.

Attwood T (1999) *Asperger's syndrome*. Jessica Kingsley Publishers, London.

Attwood T (2008) *The Complete Guide to Asperger's Syndrome*, Jessica Kingsley Publishers, London.

Attwood T (ed) (2014) *Been There, Done That, Try This! An Aspie Guide to Life on Earth*, Jessica Kingsley Publishers, London.

Baird G, Simonoff E, Pickles A, Chandler S, Loucas T & Charman DT (2006) 'Prevalence of disorders of autism spectrum in a population cohort of children in South Thames', *Lancet*, 368(9531), pp 210–215.

Baron-Cohen S (2008) *Autism and Asperger Syndrome*, Oxford University Press, Oxford.

Bejerot S, Eriksson J, Bonde S, Carlstrom K & Eriksson MBE (2012) 'The extreme male brain revisited: gender coherence in adults with autism spectrum disorder', *The British Journal of Psychiatry*, 201(2), pp 116–123. doi:10.1192/bjp.bp.111.097899.

Bejerot S, Eriksson J, (2014) 'Sexuality and gender role in autism spectrum disorder: A case control study'. *PLoS One*, **2014** - journals.plos.org

Bogdashina O (2016) *Sensory Perceptual Issues in Autism and Asperger Syndrome*: 2nd Edition: Jessica Kingsley Publishers, London.

Brownlow LC (2015) 'Investigating interoception and body awareness in adults with and without autism spectrum disorder', *Autism Research*, 8 (6), pp 709–716.

Bulluss E & Sesterka S (2020) 'When a late diagnosis of autism is life changing'. Retrieved from https://www.psychologytoday.com/us/blog/insights-about-autism/202001/when-late-diagnosis-autism-is-life-changing/.

Cassidy S, Bradley P, Robinson J, Allison C & Baron-Cohen MS (2014) 'Suicidal ideation and suicide plans or attempts in adults with Asperger's syndrome attending a specialist diagnostic clinic: a clinical cohort study', *The Lancet Psychiatry*, 1(2), pp 142–147.

Coleman-Smith RS, Smith R, Milne E & Thompson AR (2020) 'Conflict versus congruence: a qualitative study exploring the experience of gender dysphoria for adults with autism spectrum disorder', *Journal of Autism and Developmental Disorders*. 50:2643–2657.

Dalton KM, Nacewicz BM, Johnson T, Schaeper HS, Gernbacher MA, Goldsmith HHJH, Alexander AL & Davidson EJ (2005) 'Gaze fixation and neural circuitry of face processing in autism', *Nature Neuroscience*, 8, pp 519–526.

Desaunay P, Briant AR, Bowler DM, Ring M, Garardin P, Baylete JM, Guénolé F, Eustache F & Parienti JJ (2019) 'Memory in autism spectrum disorder: a meta-analysis of experimental studies', *Psychological Bulletin*, 146(5), pp 371–410. doi:10.1037/bul0000225.

Drew G (2017) *An Adult with an Autism Diagnosis: A Guide for the Newly Diagnosed*, Jessica Kingsley Publishers, London.

Eriksson SJM (2014) 'Sexuality and gender role in autism spectrum disorder: a case control study', *PLoS One*, 9(1), pe87961. doi:10.1371/journal.pone.0087961.

Gardner RM, Dalman C & Lee DBK (2020) 'The association of paternal IQ with autism spectrum disorders and its comorbidities: a population-based cohort study', *Journal of the American Academy of Child and Adolescent Psychiatry*, 59(3), pp 410–421.

Garfinkel SN, Tiley C, O'Keeffe S, Harrison NA & Critchley AKHD (2016) 'Discrepancies between dimensions of interoception in autism: implications for emotion and anxiety', *Biological Psychology*, 114, pp 117–126.

Geurts AH (2016) 'Psychiatric co-occurring symptoms and disorders in young, middle aged and older adults with autism spectrum disorder', *Journal of Autism and Developmental Disorders*, 45(6), pp 1916–1930.

Grandin T (2006) *Thinking in Pictures*, Bloomsbury Publishing, London.

Grandin T (2013) The Autistic Brain, Rider, Elbury Publishing, London

Hendrickx S (2015) *Women and Girls with Autism Spectrum Disorder: Understanding Life Experiences from Early Childhood to Old Age*, Jessica Kingsley Publishers, London.

Hirvikoski T, Mittendorfer-Rutz E, Boman M & Lichtenstein HP (2016) 'Premature mortality in autism spectrum disorder', *The British Journal of Psychiatry*, 208(3), pp 232–238.

Howlin P, Goode S & Rutter JM (2004) 'Adult outcomes for children with autism', *Journal of Child Psychology and Psychiatry*, 45, pp 212–229.

Huke V, Turk J, Saeidi S & Morgan AJF (2013) 'Autism spectrum disorders in eating disorder populations: a systematic review', *European Eating Disorders Review: The Journal of the Eating Disorders Association*, 21(5), pp 345–351.

Jackson L (2002) *Freaks, Geeks and Asperger Syndrome*, Jessica Kingsley Publications, London.

Kanner L (1943) 'Autistic disturbances of affective contact', *Nervous Child*, 2, pp 217–250.

Kim C (2013) *I Think I Might Be Autistic: A Guide to Autism Spectrum Disorders and Self Diagnosis for Adults*, Narrow Gauge Press, USA.

King JB, Prigge MBD, King CK, Morgan J, Dean DC, Freeman A, Vilaruz JAM, Kane KL, Bigler ED, Alexander AL, Lange N, Zielinski BA, Lainhart JE & Anderson JS (2018) 'Evaluation of differences in temporal synchrony between brain regions in individuals with autism and typical development', *JAMA Network Open*, 1(7), pe184777. doi:10.1001/jamanetworkopen.2018.4777.

King MD, Fountain C & Bearman DP (2008) 'Estimated autism risk and older reproductive age', *American Journal of Public Health*, 99(9), pp 1673–1679.

Kolevzon A & Reichberg RA (2007) 'Prenatal and perinatal risk factors for autism', *Arch Pediatric Adolescent Medicine*, 161(4), pp 326–333.

Lawson W (2019) *Dr. Wenn B. Lawson*. Retrieved from https://www.wennlawson.com.

Ledgin N (2002). *Asperger's and Self-Esteem*, Future Horizons, Arlington, TX.

Lipsky K (2011) *From Anxiety to Meltdowns*, Jessica Kingsley Publishers, London.

Lord C, Luyster RJ, Gotham K & Guthrie W (2012) 'Autism Diagnostic Observation Schedule, Second Edition (ADOS-2)', Western Psychological Services.

Lugnegårda T & Gillberg MUC (2012) 'Personality disorders and autism spectrum disorders: what are the connections?', *Comprehensive Psychiatry*, 53(4), pp 333–340.

Mahler K (2015) Interoception: The Eight Sensory System, Shawnee Mission, KS, AAPC, 2015

Murray D, Lesser M & Lawson W (2005) 'Attention, monotropism and the diagnostic criteria for autism', *Autism*, 9 (2). https://doi.org/10.1177/1362361305051398

National Autistic Society (2016) 'Employment survey – the National Autistic Society'.

Nomi JS & Uddin IL (2019) 'Insular function in Autism', *Progress in Neuro-Psychopharmacology and Biological Psychiatry*, 89, pp 412–426.

Ohlsson Gotby V, Lichtenstein P, Langstrom N, Pettersson E (2018) Childhood neurodevelopmental disorders and risk of coercive sexual victimization - a population based prospective twin study. Journal of Child Psychology and Psychiatry, Sep; *59* (9): 957–965, doi10 1111/jcpp12884

Panek TR (2013) *The Autistic Brain*, Rider, Ebury Publishing, London.

Pecora LA, Hancock G & Stokes GM (2019) 'Characterising the sexuality and sexual experience of autistic females', *Journal of Autism and Developmental Disorders*, 49, pp 4834–4846.

Powell T & Acker L (2016) 'Adults experience of an Asperger syndrome diagnosis: analysis of emotional meaning and effect on participants life', *Focus on Autism and Developmental Disorders*, 31(1), pp 72–80.

Ramachandran VS (2011) *The Tell-Tale Brain*, William Heinemann, London.

Roelfsema M, Hoekstra R, Allison C, Wheelwright S, Brayne C, Mathews F, Baron-Cohen S (2012) Are autism spectrum conditions more prevalent in an information technology region? A school based study of three regions in the Netherlands. *Journal of Autism and Developmental Disorders*, 42(5), pp 734–739.

Santomauro J (ed) (2012) *Autism All-Stars*, Jessica Kingsley Publishers, London.

Scott F, Baron-Cohen S, Bolton P & Brayne C (2002) 'The CAST (childhood Asperger syndrome test): preliminary development of UK screen for mainstream primary-school children', *Autism*, 6(1), pp 9–31.

Seitzer M, Kraus M, Shatluck P, Orsmond G & Lord AC (2003) 'The symptoms of autism spectrum disorders in adolescence and adulthood', *Journal of Autism and Developmental Disorders*, 33(6), pp 565–581.

Silberman S (2015) *Neurotribes*, Allen & Unwin, London.

Shore S & Rastelli L (2006) *Understanding Autism for Dummies*. Wiley, New Jersey, USA.

Smith Myles B, Tapsco H, Cook K, Miller N & Robbins LL (2000) *Asperger Syndrome & Sensory Issues*, Autism Asperger Publishing Company, Shawnee Mission, KS.

Stanford A (2011) *Business for Aspies*, Jessica Kingsley Publishers, London.

Synder A & Chi SR (2012) 'Switching on creativity', *Scientific American Mind*, 22, pp 58–62.

**Thrower E, Bretherton I, Pang KC & Cheung JDAS** (2020) 'Prevalence of autism spectrum disorder and attention-deficit hyperactivity disorder amongst individuals with gender dysphoria: a systematic review', *Journal of Autism and Developmental Disorders*, 50(3), pp 695–706.

**Tromsans S, Chester V, Kiani R, Alexander R & Brugha T** (2018) 'The prevalence of autism spectrum disorders in adult psychiatric inpatients: a systematic review', *Clinical Practice and Epidemiology in Mental Health*, 14, pp 177–187.

**Treasure J** (2013) 'Coherence and other autistic spectrum traits and eating disorders', *Nordic Journal of Psychiatry*, 67(1), pp 38–42.

**Volkmar F & Pauls AD** (1998) 'Nosological and genetic aspects of Asperger syndrome', *Journal of Autism & Developmental Disorders*, 28, pp 457–463.

**Willey LH** (1999) *Pretending to Be Normal: Living with Asperger's Syndrome*, Jessica Kingsley Publishers, London.

**Williams D** (1992) *Nobody, Nowhere*, Time Books, New York, NY.

**World Health Organization** (2020) *International Classification of Diseases*: 11th Edition: World Health Organization, Geneva.

**Wylie P** (2015) *Very Late Diagnosis of Asperger Syndrome (Autism Spectrum Disorder)*, Jessica Kingsley Publishers, London.

**Xie R, Sun X, Yang L & Guo Y** (2020) 'Characteristic executive dysfunction for high-functioning autism sustained in adulthood', *Autism Research*, Wiley Online Library, pp 1–20.

**Zheng Z & Zou PX** (2018) 'Association between schizophrenia and autism spectrum disorder: a systematic review and meta-analysis', *Autism Research*, 11(8), pp 1110–1119.

**Zucker JC** (2016) *In a Different Key: The Story of Autism*, Allen Lane, London.

# Appendix 6

## *Autism diagnostic assessment*

Assessor:                                          Date:
Name:                                              DOB/Age:

## Reason for referral: (Why now? triggers?)

## Family details

Paint a thumb nail sketch of your family members ... work ... their personality and your relationship with them. Any neurodevelopmental diagnosis in the family?

## Early developmental history

How did people describe you as a baby? Milestones – walking /talking; Non-verbal communication, language development – unusual speech, use of language; Playing/sociability; Routines – sleep, eating etc.

## Relatives questionnaire (preferably to be completed by third party such as parents or older sibling)

1 Any complication in pregnancy or birth.

2 Did s/he join in playing games with other children?

3 Did s/he come up spontaneously for chat?

4 Was s/he speaking by 2 years?

5 Did s/he enjoy sports?

6 Was it important for her/him to fit in with peers?

7 Did s/he have any sensory issues around noise, light, small touch and taste?

8 Did s/he appear to notice details that others missed?

9 Did s/he tend to take things literally?

10 Did s/he spend time doing 'imaginative, role play, pretending' play with others?

11 Did s/he like to do things over and over in the same way all the time?

12 Did s/he find it easy to interact with other children?

13 Could s/he keep a two-way conversation going?

14 Did s/he have the same interests as his/her peers?

15 Did s/he have an interest that took up so much time that s/he did little else?

16 Did s/he have friends rather than acquaintances?

17 Did she bring you things she wanted to show you?

18 Did s/he enjoy joking around?

19 Did s/he have difficulties understanding the rules of polite behaviour?

20 Did s/he have an unusual memory for details?

21 Was her/his voice unusual?

22 Were people important to her/him?

23 Was s/he good at turn taking in conversation?

24 Did s/he say things that were tactless and socially inappropriate?

25 Did s/he have normal eye contact?

26 Did s/he like repetitive routines and struggle with change of plans?

27 Did s/he have any unusual or repetitive movements?

28 Did s/he care how s/he is perceived by the rest of the group?

29 Did s/he often turn conversation back to her/his favourite topic, rather than following others?

30 Did s/he lose the listener sometimes because of not explaining what s/he was talking about?

31 Did s/he have odd or unusual phrases?

32 Did teachers every time express any concerns over her/him?

33 Did you have concerns about her/his development?

**Education:** (Schools/friends/interests/bullied/prefer breaks or lessons? exams/grades)

**Work history:** (Jobs/skills/difficulties)

**Relationship history:** (Friends/what do you like doing together?/ sexual relationships)

**Present situation:** (Domestic/activities/how do you spend your time?)

**Mental health history:** (First episode, history, other diagnosis and comorbidity, risk, medication)

**Physical health history**

## Test results

1 AQ

2 Relatives questionnaire

3 ADOS

## DSM-V criteria A: evidence of difficulties with social communication and social interaction

### Criteria A1: difficulties with social initiation and responses

1 **Do you struggle to have back-and-forth, turn-taking and *reciprocal* conversations?**

  (a) Are you good at taking turns in conversation? Can you build on comments that others make?

  (b) Do you have a tendency to 'talk over' or interrupt the other person?

  (c) Have you been told that you frequently turn conversation back to yourself or your own topics of interest?

  (d) Is it possible that you tend to think more about what you want to say, rather than what the listener might want to talk about?

  (e) Do you have a tendency to get into one-sided conversations or monologues?

2 **Do you have difficulty with *small talk* or social chit-chat with others?**

  (a) Do you find that you don't enjoy small talk or social chit-chat?

  (b) Do you struggle to think of something to say to keep conversations going?

  (c) Do you struggle to see the point in superficial social chit-chat unless there is a clear discussion point, debate or activity?

  (d) Do you sometimes cope by deliberately preparing a 'scripted' conversation?

  (e) Do you have difficulty entering into a social group or initiating conversation?

3 Would you say that you had limited interest in *sharing* your experiences, interests or achievements with others?

    (a) Do you tend to share enjoyment, interests, news or achievements with other people?

    (b) Would you say that you generally lack interest in the thoughts, experiences and opinions of others and tend not to ask questions in conversation?

    (c) Do you experience and show pleasure in social interactions?

    (d) Do you tend to get excited if somebody has good news?

4 **Have people said that they sometimes struggle to follow your train of thought clearly when you are reporting or *explaining* events? Similarly, do you sometimes struggle to follow others' conversations?**

    (a) Have people told you that you have a tendency to jump from topic to topic in conversation so they can't follow what you are talking about?

    (b) Do you have a tendency to focus too much on details, rather than the overall picture?

    (c) Do you have a tendency to struggle to get to the point and summarise information?

    (d) Do you have a tendency to ask for clarification in a conversation? E.g. saying, 'can you explain what you mean?' or saying, 'sorry, you've lost me' or 'could you clarify please?'

## Criteria A2: difficulties with non-verbal communication

1 **Do you think that *your range of non-verbal* behaviours, such as eye contact, gestures, facial expression, speech intonation etc., are limited or unusual in any way?**

    (a) Do you have difficulty or discomfort with eye contact during conversation?

    (b) Do others comment that you use your hands to gesture too much or not at all?

    (c) Have you ever been told that your facial expressions are limited or inappropriate for the situation or do not match your feelings?

    (d) Have you ever been told that your speech is flat and monotonous and doesn't vary with emotions?

    (e) Have you ever been told that you have an unusual voice (e.g. too loud, soft, quick or 'jerky')?

(f) Have you ever been told that you are 'difficult to read' as you don't show emotion on your face?

2 **Do you struggle to read and** *interpret other people's non-verbal* **behaviour?**

(a) Do you sometimes struggle to recognise when someone is interested or bored with what you are saying?

(b) Do you have difficulty working out what someone is thinking or feeling just by looking at their face?

(c) Can you work out what people mean when they change their intonation pattern, for example, to indicate sarcasm?

(d) Do you have difficulty spotting if someone in a group is feeling awkward or uncomfortable?

(e) Do you have difficulty telling if someone is masking their emotions or says one thing but means another?

(f) Do you have difficulty 'reading between the lines', identifying another person's intentions?

## Criteria A3: difficulty with relationships

1 **Do you have difficulty making and maintaining** *friendships*?

(a) Do you find it difficult to make new friends?

(b) Do you find it difficult to judge how another person is feeling about you, for example, that they might want to be your friend?

(c) Would you say that you find the unwritten rules of social behaviour a mystery?

(d) Do you wish that you had more friends but don't know how to make them?

(e) Do you prefer to have just one or two friends at a time?

(f) Do you find interacting with younger or older people easier than interacting with your peers?

(g) What does being a friend mean to you? How do you know somebody is your friend?

2 **Do you enjoy joining in with** *social occasions* **or parties?**

(a) Do you tend to struggle with or avoid social occasions, such as parties or 'leaving dos'?

(b) Do you find it hard to know how to act in social situations?

(c) Do you prefer your own company and have a lower-than-average need for social interaction?

(d) If a friend calls at your house without planning or warning, would they be welcomed spontaneously?

3 **Do you have a tendency to be very *honest and straightforward*, saying things without considering the emotional impact on the listener (making a faux pas)?**

(a) Have you been told that your comments are too direct, honest or blunt?

(b) Have you been accused of 'being rude' or offending others or making tactless comments even if you didn't mean to?

(c) Do you often clash with other people because of holding strong views and finding it difficult to compromise?

(d) Do you tend to overshare with friends and strangers?

4 **Do you have good *insight into emotions* and how relationships work?**

(a) Do you have difficulty recognising your own emotions and what triggers them? What situations lead you to experience the following emotions (what are the triggers) and how do you know that you are experiencing these emotions – how do you physically feel inside?

   i Happy

   ii Afraid

   iii Anxious

   iv Angry

   v Sad

(b) Would you struggle to identify things that you do that might annoy or irritate other people?

   i Identify two things that you do that might annoy others?

   ii Identify two things that others do that annoy you?

(c) Do you struggle to describe other people's personalities? Describe the personality of your father and mother.

(d) Have you found it hard to tell if someone is teasing, mocking or taking advantage of you?

## DSM-V criteria B: restrictive repetitive patterns of behaviour, interests or activities

### Criteria B1: atypical movement and speech

1 **Do you have any** *repetitive motor mannerisms* **(e.g. hand or finger flapping or twisting) either now or in the past?**

   (a) Do you do any repetitive flapping (stimming) or flicking movements with hands or fingers or with objects?

   (b) Do you or have you in the past ever repetitively rocked, skipped, spun, walked on toes, showed complex whole-body movements or repetitively jiggled your leg?

   (c) Have you been told that you pull unusual facial expressions, grimaces or involuntary movements?

   (d) Do you ever make repetitive vocalisation, such as humming or grunting sounds?

   (e) Do you repetitively pick at your skin or scalp?

   (f) Have you ever found release or enjoyment in an activity such as banging your forehead repetitively?

   (g) Would you say that you had poor coordination, dexterity and sense of body in space? Were you poor at sports?

2 **Do you** *use objects* **in ways other than they were intended (e.g. twirling a piece of string, chewing an object, fiddling with an object)?**

   (a) Have you ever been absorbed by things that spin, such as a washing machine, a fan or wheels?

   (b) Have you ever repetitively turned lights on and off, twirled a pen in your fingers, opened or closed doors or lined up toys or objects?

3 **Do you use** *language in an, unusual, or atypical way?*

   (a) Has anybody ever said to you that your use of language is formal or overly precise (as a child speaking like an adult or 'little professor')?

   (b) Would you say that you have a preference for exact use of words or precise information? For example, will you give precise dates, such as 15th August 2019 rather than say 'last summer'.

   (c) Do you repeatedly use certain words or phrases?

   (d) Have you ever been described as pedantic, either giving too much or too little information?

(e) Do you make up words, phrases, sometimes repeat or echo jingles or particular phrases in conversation?

(f) Have you ever referred to yourself by your own name rather than saying 'I'?

## Criteria B2: rigidity, rituals, routines and resistance to change

1 **Do you have a very strong adherence to specific *routines or rituals*?**

(a) Do you have set day-to-day routines, with multiple-step sequences of behaviour (e.g. insistence on same route or food)?

(b) Do you have routines that other people think are unusual?

(c) Do you have to have things planned out in your head?

(d) Do you collect things, categorise or arrange objects in a particular way (e.g. belongings etc.)?

(e) Do you have rules that you like to follow and expect others to follow?

2 **Do you prefer to do things in the same way over and over again, struggling *with change*?**

(a) Do you like to settle into a regular routine and then see no need to change it?

(b) Do you get very upset when the way you like to do things is suddenly changed?

(c) Do you get very annoyed when possessions and belongings get moved or rearranged by others?

(d) If there is an interruption, do you struggle to switch back quickly to whatever you were doing?

(e) Do you have a tendency to watch films or a television programme over and over again?

3 **Would you say that you have a rather '*black and white*', 'all or nothing', thinking style, where there is little room for 'the middle ground' or 'shades of grey'?**

(a) Do you have a tendency to think of issues as being black and white (e.g. politics or morality) rather than considering multiple perspectives in a flexible way?

(b) Do you have a strong sense of social justice, about what is 'right or wrong', with great difficulty compromising?

(c) Do you find it difficult seeing the other person's point of view in a discussion and find it difficult to change your opinion?

(d) Do you get frustrated if things are not clearly defined? When others say, for example, 'It depends', or 'How do you feel' or ask 'open-ended questions', which seem vague?

(e) Do you find it difficult to do more than one thing at a time (multitasking)?

4 **Would you say that you have difficulty with *imagination* and tend to take things *literally*?**

(a) Do you struggle to make up a spontaneous imaginary story?

(b) Did you tend not to engage in make-believe, imaginative or pretend play as a child?

(c) Would you prefer reading (1) factual, technical, non-fiction or science fiction books as opposed to reading (2) fiction or novels about real life?

(d) Do you find it difficult recognising the implied or hidden meaning in speech (e.g. someone saying, 'You are the apple of my eye'), often missing the point, nuance or gist?

(e) Do you find it difficult recognising sarcasm, irony, jokes and certain types of humour?

## Criteria B3: intense or unusual interests

1 **Do you have all-encompassing preoccupations or *special interests* that are unusual either in intensity or focus?**

(a) Do you tend to get obsessed with certain topics that take over many aspects of your life?

(b) Do you find yourself talking, thinking or reading about it, collecting information or items or cataloguing aspects of that interest?

(c) Do you frequently get so absorbed in one thing that you lose sight of other things?

(d) Do you have interests that are very intense and narrow in focus, compared to the interests that others might have?

(e) Do you like to research and collect information about categories of things and have a large store of factual information (e.g. dates, models, types of cars, capital cities, types of birds, sports, etc.)?

(f) Do you have a desire to understand how things work, often asking the question, 'Why?' repetitively, and wanting to research and drill down into topics?

2 Do you have an *'eye for detail'* or a persistent preoccupation with noticing parts of objects or systems?

   (a) Do you find that you tend to focus on the details rather than the overall idea?

   (b) Do you have a passion for, or notice, or have a particularly good memory for car number plates, dates, numbers, passwords, telephone numbers, words or other strings of information?

   (c) Do you tend to notice patterns, details and small changes that others do not?

   (d) Do you have an unusual attachment to a particular object, which you like to have with you?

   (e) If someone moved one of your possessions in your room, even slightly, would you notice?

3 Do you consider yourself a *perfectionist* and have to get things 'just right'?

   (a) Do you have difficulty varying your own pace of work, or varying quality, or cutting corners when carrying out a task?

   (b) Do you have difficulty prioritising, deciding what the most important aspect of a task is and what is least important?

   (c) Do you have a strong need to complete or finish a task properly, before moving on?

## Criteria B4: atypical sensory experiences

1 Do you have a particular sensitivity to *noise*?

   (a) Do you find certain loud noises unusually painful and distressing (e.g. alarm, hoover, siren, drill, a baby crying etc.)?

   (b) Do you often notice small sounds that others do not notice (e.g. ticking clock, people eating or people breathing)?

   (c) Do you have difficulty following conversations when there is a lot of background noise?

2 Do you have a particular sensitivity to *touch*?

   (a) Are you unusually sensitive to any light touch on your skin?

   (b) Do you cut the labels or tags out of your clothes?

   (c) Do you find that you are overly sensitive to certain textures (e.g. wool) and dress for comfort rather than fashion?

   (d) Do you like deep pressure such as tight hugs, tight body warmers or heavy blankets?

(e) Do you only do handshakes if essential?

(f) Do you find common self-care tasks like having a shower, haircut, cutting nails, brushing teeth, etc. uncomfortable or painful?

(g) Do you particularly like to touch certain textures or find them calming? For example, a soft fidget toy or scarf?

### 3 Do you have a particular sensitivity to *light*?

(a) Do you find a certain type of intensity of light, or bright lights, (such as neon lights or bright sunlight) painful or hard to tolerate?

(b) Have you ever had a fascination with certain lights, shiny things or spinning objects?

### 4 Do you have a particular sensitivity to *taste*?

(a) Do you find it impossible to eat certain types of food because of the unpleasant taste or texture, e.g. slimy food or crunchy food?

(b) Do you separate food on your plate or eat items individually rather than mixing and/or avoid putting sauces on food?

(c) Would you say that you have a restricted diet or has anybody said that you are a fussy eater?

(d) Do you have a distinct preference for either very bland food or highly flavoured food?

### 5 Do you have a particular sensitivity to certain *smells*?

(a) Are you unusually sensitive to certain specific smells (e.g. perfume, aftershave, bleach), often to the point that if you can't escape them, you'll become physically ill?

(b) Are you strongly drawn to certain smells, textures or visual patterns?

### 6 Do you have a particular sensitivity or insensitivity to *temperature, pain, appetite* or other bodily sensations?

(a) Do you have an unusually high tolerance of pain?

(b) Are you unusually sensitive or insensitive to temperature?

(c) Are you good at noticing the early stages of bodily sensations such as if you are beginning to feel hungry, thirsty or tired?

### 7 Do you worry about sensory overload – being *overwhelmed*?

(a) Do you sometimes feel so overwhelmed by your senses that you have to isolate and shutdown or run the risk of having a 'meltdown'?

## Criteria C: symptoms present from early childhood

## Criteria D: symptoms together limit and impair everyday functioning

## Summary and conclusions

(a) Context

(b) Diagnosis

(c) Reaction to diagnosis

(d) Comorbidity/risk

(e) Strengths

(f) Future care plan and recommendation

| DSM-V Criteria | Evidence | | | |
|---|---|---|---|---|
| Criteria | None | Limited | Moderate | Significant |
| **Criteria A (three required)** | | | | |
| **A1: Difficulties with social initiation and responses** | | | | |
| **A2: Difficulties with non-verbal communication** | | | | |
| **A3: Difficulties with relationships** | | | | |
| | | | | |
| **Criteria B (two required either past or present)** | | | | |
| **B1: Atypical movements and speech** | | | | |
| **B2: Rituals, routines and resistance to change** | | | | |
| **B3: Intense or unusual interests** | | | | |
| **B.4: Atypical sensory experiences** | | | | |
| **Symptoms present from early childhood** | | | | |
| **Collateral or third party verification** | | | | |
| **Impact (work/study, social, family/ relationships, mental health)** | | | | |

# Index

Italicized and **bold** pages refer to figures and tables respectively.